# Hyperbolic Stretching

Alex Larsson

# CONTENTS

1   Hyperbolic Stretching                                   1

2   Full Body Flexibility                                   74

3   Mind Power Unleashed                                    88

4   The 8-Minute Strength & Fat Loss (HIIT to FIT)   118

# HYPERBOLIC STRETCHING

## INTRODUCTION

Dear reader,

I have created this manual with sincere effort to show you the fastest and most effective method for achieving full body flexibility and exceptionally strong pelvic floor muscles using a simple yet enormously effective stretching program.

This program is suitable for anyone, not only athletes but regular folks who needs to revitalize their muscles and get some extra mobility and elasticity.

Over the years my only passion was hiking – a passion that made my leg muscles tight and short. Yet I was able to achieve full flexibility and maximum pelvic strength. Surprisingly, pelvic floor muscles are often

neglected in training even though they are located at the center of your gravity – a spot that controls all movements, balance and coordination.

Men and women of all ages who went through the program achieved the same results as I did simply because this method is based on scientific facts and centuries of experience. Although I discovered the initial hint from an

ancient stretching routine of Japanese Sumo fighters, I have spent two years improving the routine so it can fit anyone's physiology and current physical condition. Let it be known that sumo fighters are one of the most flexible people on the planet!

What you're about to learn here works.

Positive effects and benefits of this simple stretching routine are countless.

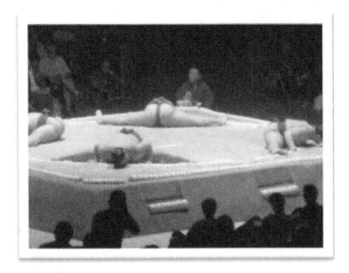

Yes, you will be able to do suspension splits like the one below easily.

The #1 rule to faster flexibility gain is to **focus on stretching your thigh muscles first**. I am talking about three muscles - the hamstrings, groin muscles (adductors) and the hip flexor (the muscle that lifts your knee up to your chest).

**If you're only interested in increasing strength of your pelvic floor muscles (without achieving splits and overall body flexibility) there is a shortened routine in one of the chapters**

**below**.

Without flexible thigh muscles your mobility, athletic skills, static yoga postures, kicking techniques and overall performance will lack high level of quality, stability, balance, speed and power.

For those who do not realize all the scientifically proven health benefits of strong pelvic floor muscles can find comprehensive list in the next chapter.

Lack of flexibility in your lower body (legs and hips) influences elasticity of other muscles as well.

For example, it is difficult to properly stretch your calves, lower and upper back or your glutes without first having flexible thighs because many postures that stretch these upper body muscles require you to have your hamstrings, adductors and hip flexors flexible as well.

With flexible thigh muscles, achieving elasticity in other parts of your body will become easier, safer and faster.

Despite this method will make your muscles highly flexible and strong, you will need to spend some energy resources to reach this objective.

You won't have to exercise in high intensity exercise fashion, but there is some muscle effort involved.

At the end of this book, I have added one chapter about warm-up exercises. Proper warm-up is gravely important for increasing your overall flexibility and for general injury prevention in training.

A good warm-up exercise will not only help you perform better in your main training or competition. It will also help you achieve better results in your main flexibility enhancement session that should be performed at the end of your main workout.

Please remember, this is a highly intelligent stretching program – not a list of new miraculous stretching positions that many hope to discover.

Just buying a book won't make you flexible. You need to go through the program to see tangible real-life results.

If you want to gain results faster and your muscles are stiff from years of inactivity or heavy weightlifting, there is no other way but to rely on sound scientific stretching exercise protocols and experiences of others.

The stretching protocol I am about to share with you is based on real-world scientific research. You will be tricking your own survival body reflexes that will accelerate your flexibility levels beyond belief.

PLEASE READ THIS MANUAL AT LEAST ONCE IN ITS ENTIRETY.

THERE ARE MANY IMPORTANT DETAILS YOU NEED TO KNOW TO MAKE THE MOST OUT OF THIS METHOD.

Plus, the stretching exercises will also totally isolate your pelvic floor muscles and make them very strong quickly – something no other method can do.

Isolating your pelvic floor muscles will help them grow. I resort the right to repeat some concepts in this book several times over where appropriate, believing this will help you understand and memorize the concepts and exercises. This will help you achieve things you have never thought were possible before.

## FULL FLEXIBILITY AND PELVIC STRENGTH

In general, stretching is still heavily underestimated discipline despite its positive effects on health and sports performance were proven in countless medical case studies. Increased muscle flexibility, especially in your thighs, hips and lower back positively impacts:

• long term emotional state and optimistic mindset

• improved athletic skills such as jump height or speed of movement

• endurance and stamina

• sexual performance and libido

• back pain health and full recovery from sciatica

• general musculoskeletal and neuro-muscular health

• overall mobility, balance, coordination and motor skills

• injury prevention and accelerated injury healing

If your bones and muscles are healthy, you can reach high degree of flexibility regardless of your age quickly and safely.

In fact, it is possible for you to achieve maximum static and dynamic flexibility including full splits in just weeks.

Increased strength of pelvic floor muscles is crucial to long-term health.

Many studies have already proven that strong and developed pelvic floor muscles can also help men and women of all ages to:

• improve bladder and bowel control (avoid urine, gas and stool leakage) in just weeks

• increase overall self-confidence and quality of life

• reduce the risk of prolapse in women and men

• in women, improve recovery from childbirth and gynecological surgery (in women)

• in men, improve long-term prostate health and recovery after prostate surgery.

• spend less muscular energy during sex and increase overall endurance in intimate moments

• in men, expose part of penis root that adds up to its length and to some degree to diameter as well

• in men, increase blood-flow in hip region during sexual activity that leads to longer and harder erections stronger orgasms in women

• in men, gain control over or delay ejaculations and increase number of orgasms men and women can have in a set time frame.

## PELVIC STRENGTH FOR JUMP & SPEED

It has been maintained for years that having strong core muscles of your abdominals and lower back significantly increases movement coordination, velocity and even the height to which you're able to jump.

Obviously, these muscles are located in the center of your gravity and thus have direct effect on your mobility.

What hasn't been publicly shared is the fact that pelvic floor muscles, also located at the center of your gravity are equally if not more important.

Why?

It's because pelvic muscles are located right at the spot where your lower body connects to your upper body with the one single muscle responsible for this connection - the hip flexor which is part of the thigh muscle family.

What few people know is that pelvic floor muscles stabilize the hip flexor this giving you even more power, speed and strength in dynamic and static movements.

As a result of this extra support from pelvic floor muscles you will experience more speed, jump height and control over your spinning and twisting movements. This is particularly beneficial to martial artists, trickers, parkour practitioners and dancers.

So if you want more mobility and don't want to get top flexibility (which you should definitely want as well) please use the simplified routine in one of the chapters below.

## WHAT RESULTS TO EXPECT

Based on results my students achieved with this method, I can confidently say that you will achieve maximum flexibility, pelvic floor strength in approximately 21 to 28 days.

Plus, if you follow this program routine to the point, you will be able to display full flexibility and splits anytime without a warm up, even if:

- You're not a top athlete or not in great physical condition

- You're over 40, 50, 60 or 70-year young

- You haven't done any sport before

- You are man or woman

- You don't have any previous stretching or training experience

- You feel that your leg muscles are too stiff or shortened

- You did a lot of heavy lifting, cycling or running in the past

- You think that your hips are too tight

- You think you are too old to achieve great flexibility

Depending on your current level of strength and flexibility, results may come even faster.

In fact, those who already worked on their pelvic floor strength, have strong legs or have achieved some level of flexibility with other method before will probably see full results faster, sometimes in just one or two weeks.

Based on your current level of flexibility you can expect to do full splits in following time frame:

•        If you are out of shape or have never exercised before, you will be able to do full splits in 28 - 30 days without a warm-up.

•        If your split test shows you are about 10 to 12 inches away from full split, you can expect to reach the flat split in 24 days with warm-up.

•        If your split test shows you are 2 – 9 inches away from full split, you can expect to reach flat splits in about 18 days with warm-up.

If you are advanced practitioner of stretching and want to do full splits without warm-up, I strongly recommend you go through the full 4-week routine anyways.

Hyperbolic stretching program is of moderate difficulty.

Depending on your current flexibility level, one session takes about 8 to 15 minutes to complete. You will have to go through the program at least three, ideally four times every week – I strongly recommend four times because the less you stretch the longer it will take you to reach full flexibility.

Here is why I recommend adding this program into your training curriculum:

•        Most people who follow regular stretching protocols will never reach full flexibility or full splits, even after years of stretching. Others will be able to do the splits after years of training, but they will only be able to do them after long stretching sessions and warm-ups.

•        After you've gone through this program and gained full flexibility in those three thigh muscles I mentioned before, you won't have to stretch them so often (with this program) because it is way easier to maintain your flexibility than to develop it. At the end of this book, I will show you incredibly simple way to maintain your lower body flexibility and splits using a simple 3-minute per week routine.

There are some conditions, exceptions and rules you need to follow.

- **Stick to prescribed exercise frequency**

In order to achieve splits in 4 weeks, you need to stick to the program and never miss a single session. You can go through the

exercises at home, in the gym or outside. There is no special equipment needed. Frequency of stretching is very important. You will have to perform this program 4 times per week. If you can't do 4 then stick to three times per week (Mo – We – Fri). Skipping stretching sessions or skipping any exercise in this program may postpone your results.

- **Stick to Safety Precautions in This Guide**

In this guide, you will also find important safety precautions that you need to consider when stretching. To start with, you should never stretch any muscle past certain pain point. Light muscle pain in a stretched muscle is fine (just like in strength training) but huge pain should be avoided. Plus, if you are recovering from muscle injury, you need to either completely stop stretching until the muscle heals completely or do only light static relaxed stretching routine that is also part of this guide.

- **Flexibility Maintenance**

As I said above, the moment you are happy with your flexibility level, you can stop using the program and resort to flexibility maintenance routine. The maintenance routine only takes about 3 minutes to complete and you will have to go through it only 2 times per week.

You can focus on stretching other muscles. Of course, you can also continue the program and increase strength and flexibility further – decision is up to you.

## Morning Stiffness – An Exception to Full Flexibility Display

In the first 60 minutes after you wake-up, your flexibility is at its lowest point. As you were sleeping, blood circulation in your body decreased and your neuromuscular mechanism switched all your muscles to a "stand-by" mode by shortening them.

Within this time frame, you may not be able to do splits without some form of warm-up. As you start moving again, your blood flow increases.

Your muscles quickly get back into an 'active' state.

So, after about 60 minutes, you will be able to display your full flexibility easily without a warm-up.

**With that being said, let's zoom in on the theory and principles.**

> ### KEY TAKEWAY
>
> *Focus on increasing flexibility of your hamstrings, adductors and hip flexors first because these muscles are often involved in all other exercises that stretch other muscles, such as calves, glutes or lower and upper back. Having these thigh muscles flexible first will also help you perform advanced dynamic movements found in*

## YOUR OBJECTIONS CLEARED

Many people haven't reached their full flexibility potential just because they didn't use the right method of stretching. I am not here to bash other methods as I respect all types of stretching and programs – all have their benefits and drawbacks – but the key is doing something for you body on a regular basis.

I am 100% convinced that this method works on everyone and the only way to find out how well it works for you is go through the program.

I am sure there will be many objections and people trying to find theoretical reasons why the program doesn't work without even trying it out.

Before we get into the program itself, give me a moment to raise few common objections to stretching in general and answer them right here.

**Objection 1: "Maybe I am too old and my muscles are not so elastic as they used to be. Will I still be able to gain flexibility quickly."**

Yes. Even though, in advanced age your joints and tendons may lack necessary amount of collagen and thus be less responsive to stretching, they don't need to be stretched at all because....

Your muscles are already flexible enough to do the splits, right now!

What needs to be overcome is the neuromuscular contraction reflex (myotatic reflex) that prevents full flexibility display.

Everything is explained in this book. If you are still in doubt, do the split test explained in the next chapter.

**Objection 2: "My muscles are too stiff from previous heavy weight lifting to be able to make them flexible again."**

While it is true that low repetition weight lifting creates muscular micro- tears that heal at shorter length, this does not mean you won't be able to reach full flexibility. Quite the opposite.

Each muscle can be stretched up to 130% of its resting length while resting in human body. In order to do splits, your muscle only needs to stretch to 105% - 108% of its normal length.

In fact, the extra muscle strength you have gained from previous resistance training may help you reach your flexibility potential much faster since strength and flexibility are closely related, as you will soon see.

If you are still in doubt, do the split test explained in my next chapter.

**Objection 3: These stretches are too simple, nothing I cannot google out or find on the web**

Yes, they indeed are googleable and they are highly effective. BUT only when they are used in combination with hyperbolic stretching protocol that you can't google out.

These stretches were carefully selected and tested following the

S.A.I.D. exercise principle explained in one of the chapters below.

As I said previously, there are no magical stretches or postures that will make you super-flexible quickly. Real magic of speed stretching lies in the exercise protocol that represents the core of this program.

**Objection 4: Yoga stretches are better**

Yoga stretches are amazing.

However, it may take years to achieve your full flexibility potential using Yoga stretches only.

If your main discipline is Yoga, then add this stretching program at the end of your yoga workout.

You will see your lower body flexibility increase dramatically in just weeks. This will in turn help you progress in your Yoga exercises faster.

**Objection 5: When I first started stretching, I felt slight hip and muscle soreness the day after. Is it dangerous?**

No, it's not dangerous. You may initially feel slight soreness in your muscles and in your hip region after your first or second stretching session.

This soreness usually comes from muscular tissue or hip tendons that have been stretched beyond their normal range of motion.

The soreness may also originate in your glutes (muscles in your buttock) that you normally don't use but they were subconsciously tensed, stretched and overloaded during your initial stretching sessions.

The hip soreness can be compared to sore muscles after your first weight lifting session. It is normal and should completely disappear in just a few days. This stretching method also counts with the soreness, so there is a solution to this issue, implemented right within this stretching program.

**Objection 6: I don't think that everyone can become flexible or do splits. What if my hips won't let me go so deep? Check online for different physiological hip formations in humans. You will see vast differences.**

Everyone should be able to do full front split with the hyperbolic stretching routine.

With side split there is one hip condition that may cause you difficulty in achieving a flat one (the one with toes pointing up).

Hip condition that may cause difficulties in achieving full straddle split is called coxa vara (see image below). However, less than 1% of the world's population have this condition.

You can easily test if you have the potential to achieve full front and straddle splits by taking the simple test below.

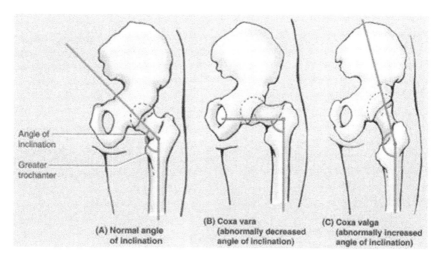

Angle of inclination

Greater trochanter

(A) Normal angle of inclination

(B) Coxa vara (abnormally decreased angle of inclination)

(C) Coxa valga (abnormally increased angle of inclination)

Coxa vara means that you have abnormally decreased angle (less than 135°

angle – image B) between neck and shaft of the femur.

However even in this case it's possible to achieve full split by tilting your pelvis, knees and toes forward. Meaning you can do a full split with toes pointing forward even if you have from this condition.

Do the test outlined below to test your split potential. If you pass the test, you will be able to do all splits easily in just a few weeks.

## THE SPLIT TEST

If you are still in doubt and think that you may not be able to achieve full flexibility potential and splits due to stiff muscles or deformed hips, do this simple test.

To test your potential for front split, take a deep lunge.

As you can see on the left image, angle between woman's left hamstring and front thigh of the rear leg is less than 180 degrees.

This means that her hip flexor will need some stretching of surrounding hip ligaments in order to achieve 180-degree angle that is required to make a nice flat front split (see image on the right).

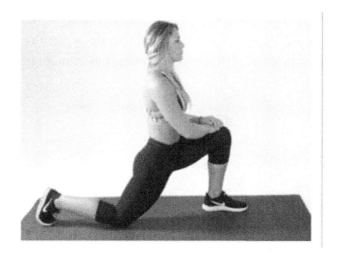

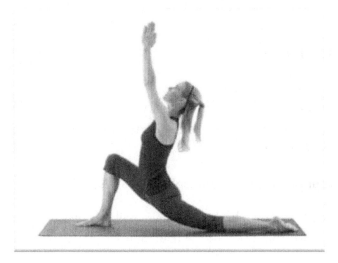

To test your potential for straddle or side split do this test.

Put one of your legs into a position as seen on the image below.

Keep your toe pointing upward. If you can keep 90-degree angle between the leg and your trunk, the only thing preventing you from doing a full split is the reflexive tension of groin muscles in both legs.

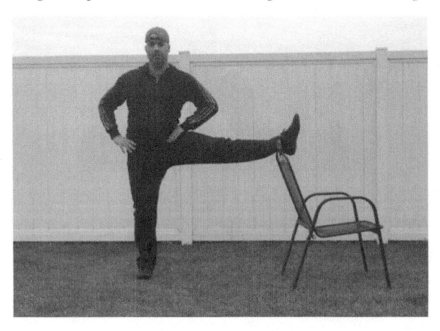

If you can do the split with one leg only, there is no deformation or muscle in your hip region that would prevent you from doing a full straddle split with both legs.

In general, it is easier to do the split with toes, knees and pelvis pointing forward than to do the straddle split with toes pointing up simply because you are using your upper body weight to gain an extra inch in the stretch.

Plus, there is no significant difference between the split with toes pointing up or toes point forward in terms of hip alignment.

The only thing that is different is that you are pointing your knees, toes and pelvis forward while arching your back to remain upright (in the split with toes pointing forward).

## THINGS TO AVOID FOR MAXIMUM FLEXIBILITY

If you perform short range movements in your sport discipline such as cycling, skating, running or even long-distance walking, always include this hyperbolic stretching program at the end of your main workout.

It has been confirmed that highly intense activities (short sprints, low repetition weight lifting etc.) slightly damage connective tissue that can in turn significantly decrease overall flexibility in just a few months if you don't do any stretching at all.

Same rule applies here.

Always do this stretching program at the end of your main workout.

Yoga stretches and exercises (asanas) are basically a form of static relaxed type of stretching where you hold certain position over extended periods of time, trying to naturally decrease the muscle tension produced by your neuromuscular system. position focus on holding relaxed muscles in a position just short of pain and reflexive muscle contraction.

When you do yoga or any form of static relaxed stretching bear in mind two important aspects that will help you make faster progress. First, to gain flexibility faster using relaxed stretching bear in mind it's a game of millimeters.

Lear how to breathe properly and deeply, and with every breath try to gain extra millimeter in the stretch.

It is a curious claim maintained by several scientists as well as most yoga masters who believe that people whose minds are not able to adapt to new situations usually are physically stiff as well. I do not share the same belief and think that this is a way too general claim.

## THE SCIENCE OF STRETCHING

I had to rewrite this chapter several times over because I didn't want to bore you to death with deep scientific explanations. Yet I wanted to give you an accurate look on why this stretching method yields results so fast.

## WHAT DETERMINES YOUR FLEXIBILITY

Let's talk about muscles, joints, tendons and ligaments.

Muscles consist of muscle fibers or cells that are parallelly aligned – just like a bundle of cords. You can contract any muscle to 65% of its length in normal resting length and you can stretch it to 130% of its normal length.

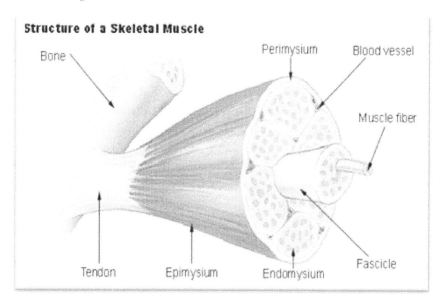

This is an important information because if a muscle can be stretched to 130% of its normal length now, it means your muscle doesn't need any more stretching in order to splits or display its full flexibility potential right now!

In other words, the reason for stretching is not to elongate the muscle but

to erase the tension in stretched muscles.

Muscles are encased in a connective tissue (epimysium) that covers all muscle fibers and connects to bones on each side of the muscle.

The hardened parts of connective tissue on both ends of every muscle are called tendons.

Tendons and connective tissue consist of collagen fibers that are strong but have its elasticity decreases after you reach 20 years of age.

That is why I suggest not to go beyond certain point of pain in your flexibility exercises. You need to protect your tendons and keep them strong.

**Ligament and joint flexibility can only be increased in young children whose muscles do not contract that much as muscles of adults. That is why you should be careful when following stretching advice from people who have gymnastic or ballet background from their childhood years. Their stretching advice may not work for you.**

Over years, collagen fibers tend to become rigid, so you want to keep that in mind. Good news is that in order to perform full splits or high kicks you

don't need to stretch your ligaments or joints at all.

Your muscles, ligaments and joints are already flexible enough for you to do the splits right now. Yes, there is no need to make your muscles more flexible than they already are.

So why can't you do splits or display maximum flexibility right now? The secret lies in muscle tension your neuromuscular system activates every time you stretch your muscles beyond its normal stretch range. Reduce the muscle tension and you'll be able to display your full flexibility potential very soon.

## REDUCING MUSCLE TENSION

Whole idea of this method is not to perform stretching exercises to make muscles more flexible but to reduce tension in those muscles by developing a new neuromuscular reflex.

Once developed, this reflex will enable you to do splits without any prior warm-up routine.

Let me give you precise insight into what happens in your body after your muscles stretch beyond its natural (daily) length. There are two crucial survival reflexes in your body that regulate muscle flexibility and muscle tension.

## MYOTATIC REFLEX

Length of your muscles is controlled by muscle fiber tension at any given time. This tension is regulated by your neuromuscular system.

In fact, there is a constant unconscious exchange of information between your muscles and your nervous system.

When your stretch a muscle beyond its normal stretch range, special sensors located in your muscle belly called 'muscle spindles' send alert to your neuro-muscular system (located in spinal cord) that in turn contracts the muscle to either prevent complete muscle tear or to keep you in balance.

Muscle spindles (see image below) are string-like sensors that extend when muscle is stretched, causing an impulse sent to your neuromuscular system. Some spindles only react to magnitude of muscle stretch while others react to both, magnitude and speed of the stretch.

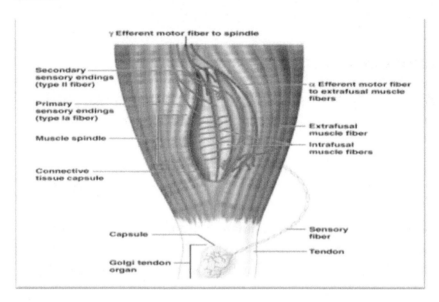

In other words, when muscle is stretched beyond its normal length, it is automatically contracted because your nervous system thinks "oh, this muscle is being stretched too far. I'd better contract that muscle before it gets totally torn apart" or "oh, this guy just slipped on a banana. I'd better contract that muscle, so he or she can regain his or her balance."

**This is the myotatic or stretch reflex also known as reciprocal inhibition.**

It is the main problem preventing you from reaching your full flexibility potential quickly and displaying it right now.

Luckily, there is also an opposite neuromuscular reflex called "autogenic inhibition reflex" that your body will use to accelerate your flexibility gains–it is also the key reflex that will let you display full body flexibility without a warm-up.

**This opposite reflex you want to take advantage of is called autogenic inhibition reflex or reversed myotatic reflex.**

## AUTOGENIC INHIBITION REFLEX

Autogenic inhibition (AI) reflex is a sudden relaxation of a muscle in response to excess tension. This automatic lengthening reflex is controlled by the central nervous system and regulated by the proprioceptors located in the tendons, mostly by the Golgi tendon organs (GTOs, see image on previous page).

A Golgi tendon organ is yet another stretch receptor that signals the amount of force developed by a muscle. The AI reflex is activated when the Golgi organ senses too much force is being applied against a muscle and tendon in static position.

Think of someone doing a bench press of weight they could not push up. Eventually the muscles basically give up and "relax." They simply turn off because if those muscles continued resisting the force, they would eventually tear down.

When this mechanism doesn't have time to take place it results in a rupture of the muscle, for example an Achilles tendon rupture that sounds like a shotgun when it tears.

How to use this information to increase your flexibility? Let's have a second look into what happens in your muscle when it is stretched. When you assume your maximum stretch position, myotatic reflex takes over immediately and contracts your muscle to prevent further stretch.

About 7 or 8 seconds later, after the myotatic reflex contracted your stretched muscle, autogenic inhibition reflex naturally takes over. Because your neuromuscular system sees no danger that your muscle is going to get torn from overstretching it will slightly relax your already stretched muscles.

However, this reflexive relaxation is not significant because muscle tension is not maximal, meaning that only some muscle fibers experience relaxation while others stay tensed.

Now, if you consciously tense (contract) the stretched muscle as much as you can, you will induce deeper inroad into muscle fibers and more of them get recruited and relaxed, helping you stretch a little further, beyond your initial maximum stretch.

Repeat this conscious tension several times over and you will be able to relax more muscle fibers and go deeper into the stretch. If you want to be able to relax substantial amount of muscle fibers using autogenic inhibition reflex, much powerful conscious muscle tensions are required.

In order to develop intense tensions, you need to strengthen these muscles.

Once your muscles become stronger using simple strength exercises outlined in this book, the amount of recruited fibers multiplies and your body's ability to completely relax all muscle fibers will dramatically increase.

That in turn will increase your flexibility and reprogram your muscle reflexes in such a way that you will be able to display your full flexibility potential without warm-up.

In other words, the more you repeat these contractions as you progress through the routine in coming weeks, the stronger AI reflex you will develop. Eventually only one single short contraction will be necessary for you to display your full flexibility potential.

**The science behind fast flexibility gains lies in tricking your neuromuscular mechanism to change some of your natural muscle survival reflexes.**

## ONLY THREE MUSCLES

You only need to focus on stretching and tensing three muscle groups to be able to do full splits, display your full lower body flexibility and grow strength in your pelvic muscles.

For front split, it's the hamstring (bicep femoris) and the hip flexor (psoas) muscle. Contrary to what you may have heard, stretching your calves is not necessary for achieving full front split.

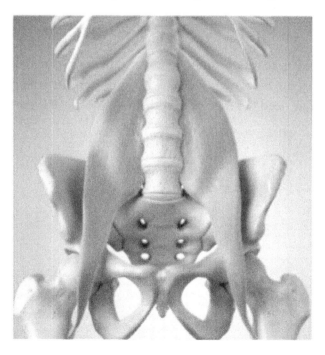

Image above shows the iliopsoas muscle, the strongest hip flexor in human body. There is no need to strengthen this muscle as it is already strong enough for our purposes.

Its main function is to keep your posture, move your legs forward and pull your knees up to your chest.

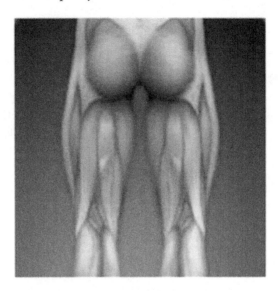

Image above is the hamstring. Its main function is knee flexion and extension of the hip when the trunk is fixed. For side split or straddle split you only need to stretch the adductors. That's all there is to it.

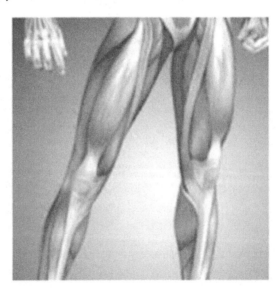

All three muscles reside in your thighs (the hip flexor only partially). Once you achieve flexibility in these muscles and resort to the 3-minute leg flexibility maintenance routine, you can focus on increasing flexibility in other muscles, important to your specific training discipline. For example, lower and upper back muscles, arms, chest, glutes or calves.

## THE HYPERBOLIC STRETCHING ROUTINE

The Hyperbolic Routine is very simple although demanding on muscle strength, for reasons specified above.

The whole routine should take no more than 15 minutes to complete (not counting the warm-up session).

If you plan to do this routine as a standalone set, here is how it should look like:

•       Warm Up Joint Rotation (1 minute)

•       Aerobic activity, i.e. skipping rope, jumping jacks etc. (5 minutes)

•       Static relaxed stretches to warm up (5 minutes)

•       Flexibility-specific strength training (8 minutes)

•       Hyperbolic Stretching (12 minutes)

If you do this routine as part of some specific training (yoga, martial arts, dancing, weightlifting etc.), here's the breakdown:

•       Joint rotations

•       5 minutes of aerobic warmup (skipping rope, shadowboxing etc.)

•       Static stretching specific to your discipline

•       Your main training session (yoga, martial arts, dancing etc.)

•       Heavy weightlifting routine or strength training

- Flexibility-specific strength exercises

- Hyperbolic stretching

Hyperbolic stretching is always performed after your normal training session (i.e. MMA, martial arts, yoga, ballet, weightlifting etc.) as part of your post training cool-down.

Hyperbolic stretching should never be performed as part of a warm-up before your regular training, as it can quickly fatigue your muscles, making your main training session less effective and risky in terms of possible injury.

If you need to display full static flexibility during your main training session, do 5 minutes of aerobic activity followed by simple static and dynamic stretches in your warm-up.

Never do hyperbolic stretching more than four times per week. Your muscles need enough recovery time since the routine is demanding on your muscle fibers. Detailed routine breakdown now follows.

## THE WARM-UP INTRO

I will go into warm-ups later but remember to always start every session with simple joint rotations.

Your joints need to be relaxed and loosened before you get them involved in strenuous activity. If you sense any pain or blockage in your joints, it is advised not to continue and see your doctor.

I haven't included joint rotation images into this book since almost

everyone knows how to do them.

Do 5 to 10 reps on either side in following progression. Wrists, elbows, whole arms, neck, upper body, hips, knees and finally the ankles.

This should be followed by 5 minutes of aerobic activity and light static stretches that will prepare you for the main training session.

## FLEXIBILITY-SPECIFIC STRENGTH ROUTINE

Improving muscle strength of stretched muscles is very important part of your flexibility training. Without this strength training part, you won't be able to achieve full splits so quickly.

As I said before, the stronger your stretched muscles, the more tension you can generate in the static stretches.

As your muscle strength increases from training to training, you will see greater gains in your flexibility literally on daily basis.

How long should you do these strength exercises?

I suggest you do them for the whole duration of this program. When you reach full splits or flexibility you are happy with, you may stop doing the strength exercises and only do the quick flexibility maintenance routine two times per week.

This maintenance routine does not require you to do any strength exercises and only relies on the strength you develop using the static stretches.

However, if you want to take your flexibility into another level and want to be able to:

•       walk out from your splits without using your arms for support

- or increase your leg flexibility beyond splits

- be able to do suspension splits on two chairs…

…then you should consider continuing with the strength exercises for at least two or three more weeks to make your adductors and hamstrings even stronger.

We will only focus on strengthening the hamstrings and adductors. The hip flexor does not need to be strengthened as it is already strong enough, since you use this muscle frequently every time you move.

You can choose from three alternatives of this strength routine, depending on where you are and what equipment you have at your disposal. Do these exercises slowly and focus on keeping constant tension in the trained muscle.

**Gym Alternative**

If you're in the gym I highly suggest you use strength machines and do at least 2 sets of 30 repetitions per set. Rest about 45 seconds between each set. Select weight that will make you feel a slight muscle burn during last few reps of each set. Do not do any forced reps, do not increase resistance.

The idea here is not to destroy these muscles, just to strengthen them with low weight resistance. Always try to add few more reps in your next training session using the same weight load. Select lighter weight and Do between 30 to 40 reps.

**Exercise 1: The Hamstring Curl**

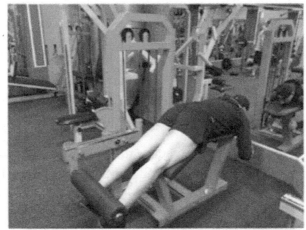

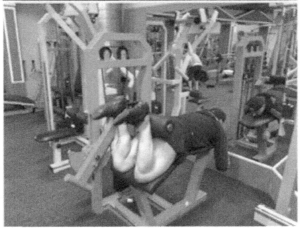

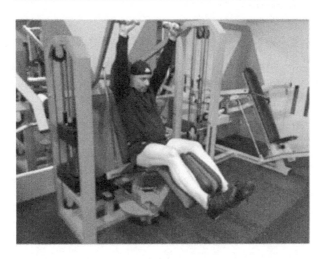

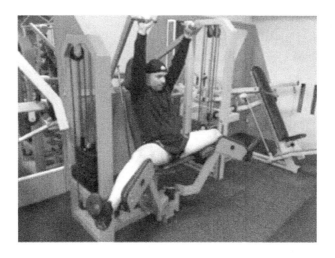

Remember to always select proper weight or proper repetition speed that will let you feel very slight burning sensation at the end of each set within the prescribed repetition range.

## Ankle Weights Alternative

If you're training outside or at home, I suggest you get a pair of ankle

weights. Each ankle weight should weigh at least 4.5lbs each.

If you can get a pair of 10lbs each, that's even better because you won't

have to do so many repetitions to properly fatigue your muscles.

You can easily get a pair of 10lbs ankle weights for a price between $15 to

$20 at amazon.com.

Do only one set of each exercise and slowly perform as many repetitions as possible. Anywhere between 50 and 200 reps is fine.

If you do 50 reps and feel a slight muscle burn, stop the set and try to add few more repetitions in your next session, using the same weight.

## Exercise 2: Weighted Adductor Flies

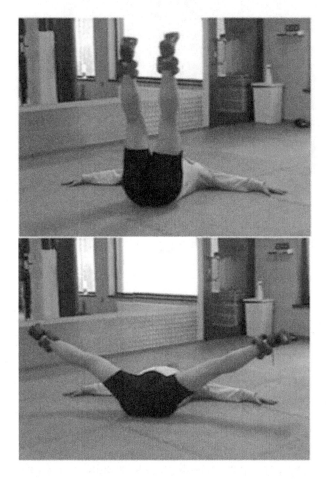

Tie up one ankle weight on each leg for the adductor flies exercise. For isolated hamstring curl you can use two ankle weights tied onto one leg to increase the resistance.

To perform isolated hamstring curl, find any kind of support and lean over it in a 30 to 45-degree angle. Straighten and secure the right leg behind the left knee. Perform slow controlled repetitions in full range of motion.

## Isolated Hamstring Curls with Ankle Weights

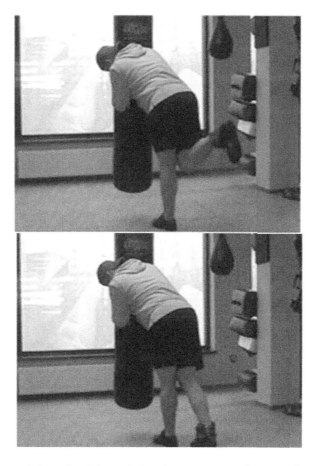

Since the weight of ankle weights is set, remember to always adjust repetition speed that will let you feel the burning sensation at the end of each set within the prescribed repetition range.

## No Equipment Alternative

If you don't want to invest into ankle weights, here is another variation you can do without any equipment. Although I'm using barbell for the squat, you can do it without any equipment and use your sheer body weight as your resistance. Spread your legs slightly more than shoulder width and do around 30 reps of wide squats. Repeat 2 times with about 45 seconds rest between sets. You can also do one long set of 50 to 200 squats if you're

well-conditioned.

Wide stance will help you put more stress on adductors and hamstrings. In order to feel muscle burn in the last few repetitions of each set you need to find appropriate the speed of movement. Slower the movement, the sooner you get the burn. In this and the next strength exercise, focus on constant muscle tension and never extend your legs completely in the top position. Never rest on the bottom position either.

**Exercise 1: Wide Squat**

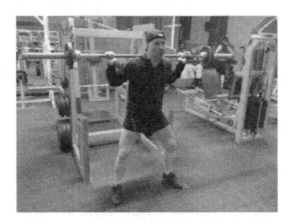

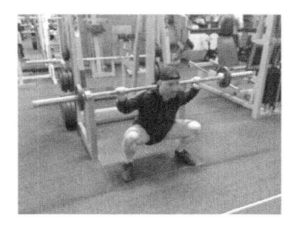

If your legs are strong, you can replace the squat with more difficult strength exercise that better targets your hamstrings and hip flexors. I am talking about front and reverse lunges.

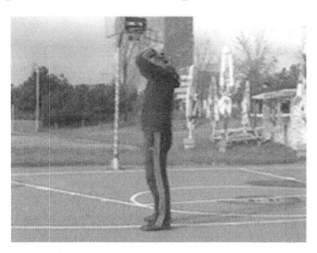

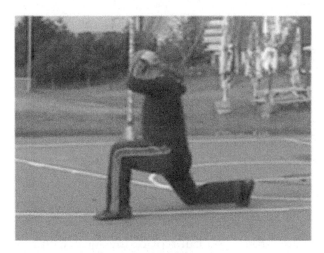

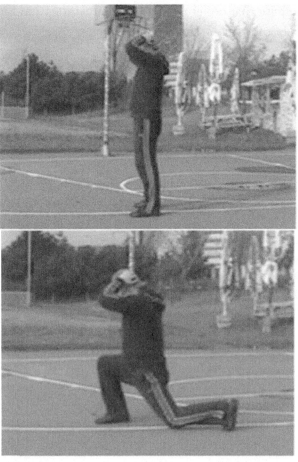

Put your palms behind your head. Take a deep lunge forward so that the knee of your rear leg touches the ground. Then step back to your original upright position. Alternate legs. Repeat as many times as it takes you to feel the burning sensation in your hamstring and hip flexor.

You can change the exercise slightly and do reverse lunges by stepping back from your upright position.

This will put a little more stress on your hip flexors.

**Exercise 2: Adductor Flies with No Weight Added**

Then, lie down on the floor and perform one long and slow set of adductor flies using sheer weight of your legs.

Do as many repetitions as it takes to feel the burning sensation in your adductors.

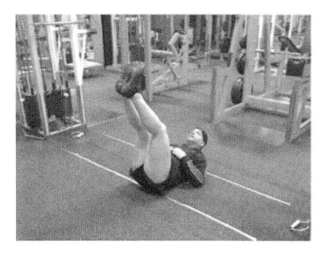

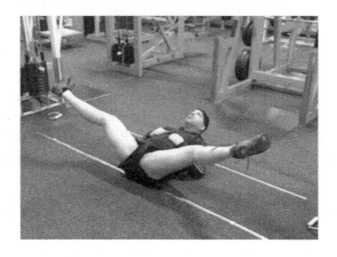

Adductor flies are done slowly, just like when you do them on the adductor machine.

Always do them in full range of motion.

Do as many reps as possible until you feel slight muscle burn. Between 50 and 200.

Reminder: Since the weight of your resistance is set (your body weight and weight of your legs) remember to always adjust repetition speed that will let you feel the burning sensation in your muscles at the end of each set within the prescribed repetition range.

After you're done with the strength part, rest one or two minutes and move

on to the hyperbolic stretching routine.

## HYPERBOLIC STRETCHING ROUTINE - WEEK 1 TO 3

Hyperbolic Accelerator Stretching is the fastest and most effective way of increasing your flexibility. It helps you overcome the muscle tension (myotatic) reflex using powerful muscle contractions that lead to increased muscle relaxation.

Hyperbolic Accelerator Stretching consists of prescribed isometric contractions and relaxations that will increase your muscle strength (including pelvic muscles) and re-train your neuromuscular system for maximum relaxation and maximum stretch.

### Exercise Selection: The SAID Principle

As you will soon discover, there are only three stretching exercises you need to perform to achieve maximum lower body flexibility and full splits.

All three exercises resemble splits themselves for a good reason. Selection of these exercises was no random event. They were selected with regards to the SAID principle.

The SAID stands for Specific Adaptation to Imposed Demands and this training principle explains that a certain exercise or type of training produces adaptations specific to the activity performed and only in the muscles that are stressed by the activity.

To go one step further, according to the SAID Principle, the body adapts in a specific fashion to the specific demands that are placed on it.

For example, if one does figure skating a lot, one will adapt to the specific skill and strength demands of figure skating (he or she will develop lower body hypertrophy, strength, explosiveness, agility, etc.).

In short, to develop a better golf swing, one should train the golf swing; to develop endurance for a marathon, one must train by running long distances.

In some instances, there is a varying degree of "cross-over," whereby adaptation from one activity will enhance traits needed to perform in another activity.

An example of this would be in training to improve grip strength directly correlates to other activities where grip strength is a requisite (pullups, deadlift, etc.). This cross-over is the reason many athletes incorporate cross-training into their programs.

This is also the same principle that drives functional training.

Recommended exercises do not fancy any strange body positioning and have been selected because you can safely and easily transfer enough weight to create muscular tension in stretched muscles – and this is what you really need if you want to achieve full flexibility quickly.

**The Stretching Exercise Protocol**

As I said in the beginning, magic of this method is in the exercise protocol.

Let me give you full explanation of what is going to happen in your body as you go through the stretching exercises.

Some of the following information has already been explained in previous chapters but I want to take it one step further.

Assume your stretching posture and stretch as far as you can.

What happens in this moment is that the myotatic reflex I spoke of earlier takes over and tenses the stretched muscle, making it impossible for you to stretch further.

When you consciously tense the already stretched muscle, reverse myotatic reflex takes place. This means your neuromuscular system will allow you to stretch a little more.

After few seconds, release the conscious tension and move about half an inch more into the stretch.

Then, tense the stretched muscle consciously again and another reversed myotatic reflex takes place.

Again, release the tension and move a bit more into the stretch. Repeat one or two more times until you achieve your maximum stretch.

What you are basically doing with the tense-relax protocol is that you're

influencing and reprogramming your neuromuscular memory system.

After few weeks your body we re-learn and replace the old tension reflex with reversed-tension reflex, making it possible to stretch all the way down to a full split.

Last thing to discuss is how long you should hold each individual tension.

## Tension-Relax Frequency and Duration

I have already explained that it is necessary to perform several tensions of the already stretched muscles in a single set and you may experience muscle cramps or shaking during the process.

Which is fine!

If your muscles shake during exercise it is because they are becoming deeply fatigued.

Normally, your body recruits exactly the number of motor units (groups of muscle fibers sharing a motor neuron) needed to produce the desired amount of force to resist a force.

As some fibers become fatigued others are recruited to take their place. Normally this happens smoothly, but the more fatigued your muscles become and the more and larger the motor units dropping out the more the force produced varies from the target and you start to shake.

So, multiple tensions and multiple sets of one stretching exercise will recruit more muscle fibers that will be prone to reprogramming.

There are two tension-relax durations you can use. Both are equally effective, however the second one is more demanding:

•        Consciously tense your already stretched muscles for 5 seconds applying about 30-40% of maximal tension. Relax for about 3 seconds and increase the stretch.

Tense the muscles again for 5 seconds, now with 50% - 60% of your maximal tension. Again, release the tension, wait for 3 seconds and try to increase the stretch. Repeat again, now with maximal tension held for 5 seconds. Then relax and increase the stretch.

Now tense again with maximum power and hold the stretch for at least 12 – 15 seconds. Your set is now over. Change legs and repeat the set. Rest about 30 seconds. Repeat at least 2 times for each leg.

•        Consciously tense your already stretched muscle and hold the tension for 10-12 seconds, applying 30% to 40% of maximal tension. Relax and increase the stretch. Repeat the 10-12 second tension two more times with 50% - 60% of your maximum and then one last time again with 100% of your maximum. Your set is now over.

Change legs and repeat the set. Rest about 30 seconds. Repeat the at least two times for each leg.

**Straddle Split Stretching Exercise (Beginner and Intermediate)**

Find any elevated flat surface where you can comfortably rest your leg. Wall bars are the absolute best for this purpose.

Your toes should be pointing forward, not up. On the images below, I am showing different flexibility levels, ranging from beginner to intermediate.

Use this exercise starting from week one up until the end of week three.

Alternatively, you can use one of the supplemental exercises as shown below. Select only one of the exercises and don't change them in the following three weeks of stretching.

In the description below, I am using the three 12-second long durations of muscle tension.

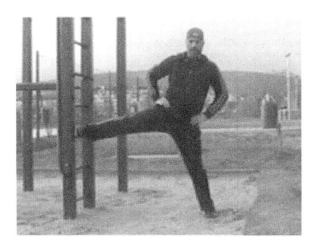

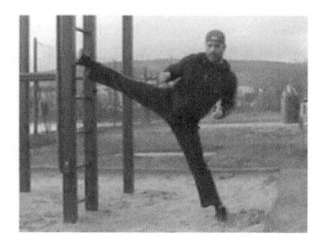

If you're new to stretching and your muscles are tight, raise your right leg low, just enough to feel the stretch (left image).

Your supporting leg should be in vertical position (90-degress in relation to the ground). Mine is little bit far away on the image.

1.      Once you assume starting position, wait about 3 to 5 seconds until your mechanisms adapt to the stretch.

2.      Now, increase the stretch as far as you can, by moving your supporting leg further away from the wall bars or elevate your leg on higher bar, or both so that will be able to keep balance.

3.      Tense your groin muscles by pushing down to the bar with your right leg and with your left supporting leg press into the ground. As if you were trying to "pinch" the space between your feet. Hold the tension for 12 seconds. Your tensions in the first week don't have to be all out. You can start at about 50% pressure and gradually increase it to maximum as your muscles get stronger. You may experience muscle cramps or shakes when you're a beginner at this point but that is exactly what you want.

4.      After 12 seconds, release the tension, relax your muscles and

try to increase the stretch by at least half of an inch, by either moving your supporting leg away from the bars or lifting your right leg higher on the next bar. Wait about 2 -3 seconds and tense your groin muscles again. Hold for 12 seconds.

5.      Repeat the tension-relaxation-stretch-tension two to three more times until you can't stretch anymore. Then change sides. This is the end of your first set.

Change sides and now lift your other leg up on the bar. Repeat. Do 2 sets for each side. That amounts to total of four sets of this exercise.

**Alternative Adductor Stretches**

Use this exercise if you have weak knees. In this position, only small portion of your body weight is transferred onto your adductors and you can regulate the amount of weight by leaning forward or backward.

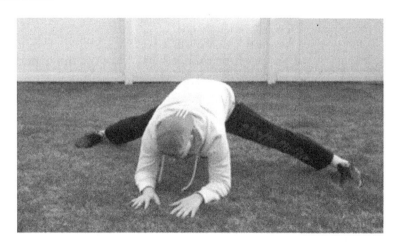

Another alternative exercise is even simpler and suitable for those who only want to strengthen their pelvic floor muscles. Again, use the same protocol – relax – increase - tense.

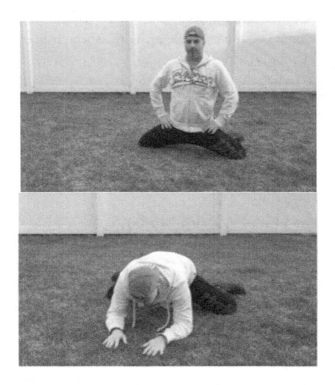

Get on your knees and spread your legs sideways as much as you can. Then, lean forward on you forearms and again, follow the hyperbolic exercise protocol. Choose only one exercise and work with it. Never combine or alternate the exercises between sessions.

**Front Split Hamstring Stretch (Beginner and Intermediate)**

After 30 seconds of rest, use the same stretching protocol but this time assume the hamstring stretch position.

Do 3 sets for each leg, totaling in 6 sets of this exercise.

Start low if you are a beginner (left image) and if you are more advanced raise your leg higher on the wall bar (right image).

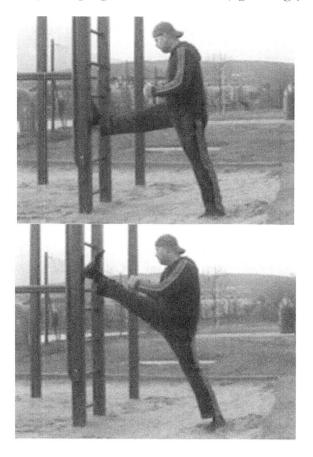

With your right leg, press down against the bar for 12 seconds.

You can also increase the tension by leaning your trunk forward over your raised leg.

Then release the tension and increase the stretch by half of an inch, by either moving your supporting leg away from the bars or raising your right leg higher on the wall bar.

Do 4 tensions, then change legs. Do 3 sets for each leg.

## Alternative Hamstring Stretch

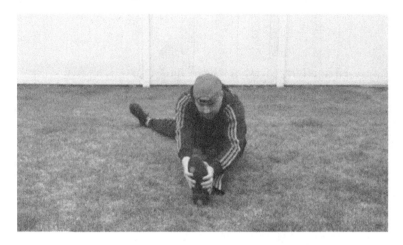

If you have any problems to use the elevated hamstring stretch, you can use the seated hamstring stretch although I believe this exercise is less efficient simply because there is no body weight that puts stress on hamstring.

Spread your legs comfortably.

Do not use your maximum spread/straddle position since we want to focus on hamstrings not adductors here.

You can even bend one of the legs or you can sit on your bed and leave one leg freely hanging from the side of your bed as you lean toward the other. Alternatively, you can even do the hurdler's stretch if you prefer.

Main point here is to apply tensions and relaxations. Lean toward the stretched leg and keep pressing your leg into the floor in order to tense your hamstring. If your back is slightly arched in the beginning that's fine.

Eventually you will be able to have your back straight and touch your knee with your chin.

## The Hip Flexor Stretch

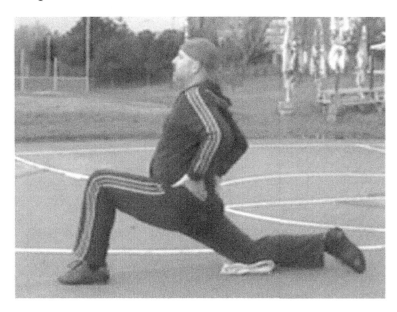

This is the last exercise. You are going to stretch your hip flexor responsible for high-quality flat front split.

Put one knee on the ground and take a long lunge forward with you other leg.

Keep your hips facing forward all the way through the exercise. This will give your hip flexor a good deep stretch.

Assume your maximum stretch posture feeling the stretch in your hip flexor.

You can increase the stretch by pushing your pelvis forward with your hands.

Now, tense your hip flexor by pressing your rear knee into the ground. Hold for 12 seconds (or apply any hyperbolic protocol mentioned above), then relax, increase the stretch and tense again.

Repeat three to five times. Change legs. Do 3 sets for each leg.

## EXERCISE FREQUENCY

For fast results, hyperbolic stretching routine should be performed ideally 4 times per week. As your flexibility increases, you may decrease session duration by decreasing the amount of sets for each stretching exercise.

Don't skip the flexibility-specific strength exercises as they will significantly accelerate your progress. Trying to increase strength only by doing the hyperbolic stretching routine is not enough for achieving splits in four weeks.

You need to do both – the strength exercises and the hyperbolic routine to achieve results fast. If your muscles hurt, reduce the intensity of tensions or stop exercising and possibly add one more day off.

However, stick to your hyperbolic stretching frequency of four times per week. If you can only do it three times per week, then go with Mo-We-Fri frequency, but bear in mind that in this case results can be delayed.

**Here's a weekly schedule you should follow:**

• Monday – Hyperbolic Stretching Routine at the end of your workout

• Tuesday - Hyperbolic Stretching Routine at the end of your workout

- Wednesday – day off

- Thursday – Hyperbolic Stretching Routine at the end of your workout

- Friday - Hyperbolic Stretching Routine at the end of your workout

- Saturday - day off

- Sunday - day off

Every hyperbolic stretching routine must be preceded by flexibility-specific low resistance/high repetition strength training routine.

## HYPERBOLIC STRETCHING ADVANCED: WEEK 4

Congratulations! If you made it past the 3-week mark, you should already see remarkable flexibility gains, feel the strength in your legs, pelvis and in your glutes.

In the fourth week, we are going to change the stretching exercises to drop you fully into all types of splits, maximize your gluteal and pelvic strength.

Maximize your contractions in every stretching session and do not forget about the strength exercises that are inevitable for achieving maximum flexibility and overall pelvic strength.

Once you get through week four, you should be able to display your maximum flexibility in your lower body.

After week four, you can resort to The Flexibility Maintenance Routine that does not involve any dynamic weight training and can be completed in less than 3 minutes.

## Straddle Split Stretching Exercise (Advanced)

Assume your maximum stretch position with the soles of your feet firmly on the ground (image below). If you want, you keep your knees slightly bent in this position to take a little weight off them.

Hold the stretch and tense your muscles using the prescribed hyperbolic protocol.

Do not touch the ground with your arms and keep balance. Your adductors and glutes should be strong enough to support you. The more complicated the stretch, the more it engraves into your muscle memory!

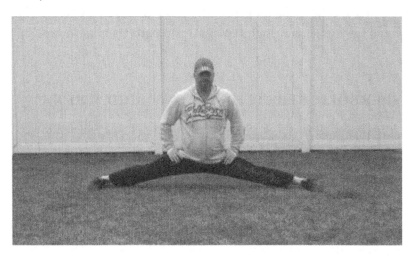

Try to increase the stretch as much as possible using 5 to 6 tensions. Don't worry about overstretching. Remember, your muscles are flexible by default. You are just activating more muscle fibers using the reverse myotatic reflex that will induce more relaxation! Do not give up!

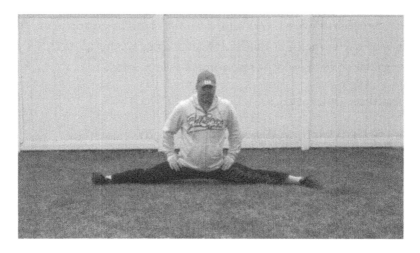

Push more to reach the full split. Eventually, you will only need one or two one-second long tensions before you will drop into a full split (see image below) without any warmup.

Hold your maximum stretch position without tension for as long as you can–minimum of 15 seconds – but you can go well over a minute for better results. I often rest in this position for one minute without any tension.

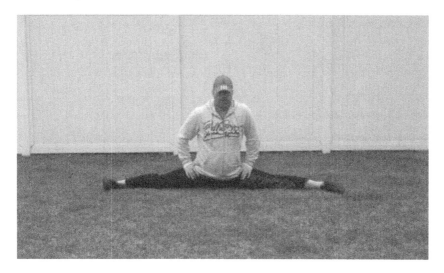

After the fourth week, you can also try the suspension split (box split) but use something that is low and close to the ground, so you have a chance to keep your balance using your arms.

Repeat three times with 30 seconds rest between sets.

**Front Split Stretching Exercise (Advanced)**

Kneel on your right knee and straighten your left leg in front of you (image below). When I stretch on hard surface, I always use knee pads.

Push the front leg forward to assume your maximal stretch position. Do not use your arms for support and keep your balance.

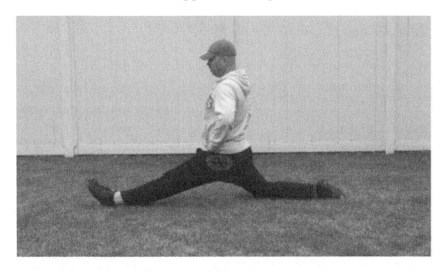

Again, use the hyperbolic stretching protocol to increase the stretch by pushing your front leg forward as much as you can.

Even if you feel you cannot do more (image below), do a few more strong tensions and push yourself further down.

Do not worry about tearing your muscles.

Your muscles are already strong enough to hold you and flexible enough for a full split!

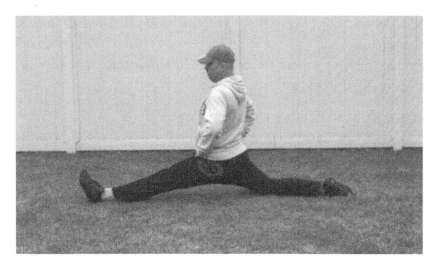

Push more to reach the full split (image below). Eventually, you will only need one or two one or two-second long tensions before you will be down in a full split (see image below) without any warm-up. Hold your maximum stretch position without tension for as long as you can – minimum of 15 seconds – but you can go well over a minute for better results.

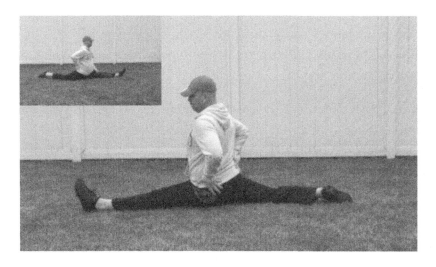

Once you get down into a full front split, you will notice that the hip of your rear leg has a tendency to turn your trunk sideways.

Try to adjust your hips so they are facing forward. This will increase the stretch in your hip flexors and let you do high quality front split with hips facing forward. Change legs and repeat three times on each side with 30 seconds rest between sets.

## WEEK BY WEEK WALKTHROUGH

It is important for you to know what to expect and what to focus on in each individual week so that you can progress quickly, safely and effectively.

### Week One

First week and your first training sessions are the most important ones in terms of motivation to get you through the entire 4-week program.

In fact, the first week should only be devoted to muscle adaptation to new stress and new training.

Since your muscles are going to experience new type of stress, new positions, tensions and load from new type of strength training, get ready to feel soreness in your muscles and hips.

Do not push yourself with muscle tensions this week. Do only mild tensions. Simply, test your new strength and stretching routine. Find your optimal weight for prescribed repetitions in your strength exercises and get used to muscle tensions while stretching your muscles.

If your first training session will be on Monday, your muscles and hips will feel sore the day after. If they don't, go through the entire session on Tuesday.

If they do feel sore, give them up to three days to recover – simply take three days off. However, since you need to complete at least four sessions every week, you need to catch up.

Your first week's routine will then look like this:

•      Monday – flexibility-specific strength training + hyperbolic stretching

•      Tuesday – day off

•      Wednesday – day off

•      Thursday – day off

•      Friday - flexibility-specific strength training + hyperbolic stretching

•      Saturday - flexibility-specific strength training + hyperbolic stretching

•      Sunday - flexibility-specific strength training + hyperbolic stretching

**Week Two and Three**

Regardless of when you have stretched the previous week, your second week's first session starts again on Monday.

In week two and three, session frequency would look like this.

•      Monday – flexibility-specific strength training + hyperbolic stretching

•      Tuesday – flexibility-specific strength training + hyperbolic stretching

•      Wednesday – day off

•      Thursday – flexibility- strength training + hyperbolic stretching

•	Friday - flexibility-specific strength training + hyperbolic stretching

•	Saturday - day off

•	Sunday - day off

In weeks two and three you should focus on proper form and a feeling of slight burn in your strength exercise sets, on increasing your stretches and tension intensity in every stretching exercise.

## Week Four

In week four you will still be stretching on Monday, Tuesday, Thursday and Friday while giving your muscles enough time to recover in the off days.

This week's primary aim is to get you down into full splits by implementing

new stretching exercises (splits).

Once you're done with week four, you should be able to display your full flexibility and splits, even without the warmup.

Plus, you should also have achieved your maximum pelvic floor and gluteal strength.

At this point you can move on to The Flexibility Maintenance Routine.

## Troubleshooting

Some people have claimed that they were still missing about an inch to a full split at the end of week four.

Reason for that is that many people do not follow the stretching frequency (four times per week) or they only stretch but don't do the strength exercises.

If you followed the routine to the point and still miss and inch to reach a full split, I suggest stop doing the strength exercises completely in the next week an only do the hyperbolic stretches. This will take a little stress of your muscles and they should be able to relax completely in the next seven days.

# LIGHT WARM UP STRETCHING

There has been a lot of confusion about which type of stretching exercises are best for proper warm up.

Some people only recommend doing dynamic stretches if your sport requires dynamic movements (i.e. kicks) as they stimulate different kind of muscle spindles in your muscles and there is a lot of science behind it.

Dynamic flexibility is a little different than static flexibility and static stretches tend to decrease blood flow in your muscles taking your mood down or away from the main training session.

Others say the best way is to combine static and dynamic exercises, while yet another group only recommends static stretches for warm-ups.

It is my personal experience that after initial joint rotations and 5 to 10 minutes of aerobic activity static stretching routine should follow.

After this part of warm-up, do few rounds of kicks or other movements, gradually increasing the speed and height.

I highly advice you master the Full Body Stretching Routine in the other manual that is part of this book. It can be used in your warm-up to prepare all your main muscles for advanced movements or as a relaxed stretching exercise at the end of your workout.

However, if you are in a hurry and do not want to learn the new warm-up stretching techniques, you can use the same stretches for warm-up as you do in the Hyperbolic Stretching routine at the end of your workout.

The only thing that changes is the exercise protocol. No tensions should be done in your warm-up stretching session. Here's the simple routine:

**Elevated Adductor Stretch**

Raise your leg on the wall bar and feel the stretch in your adductors. Try to increase the stretch every 10 seconds without consciously tensing them.

Keep them relaxed as much as you can After about 30 – 40 seconds change legs. Repeat 2 times for each leg.

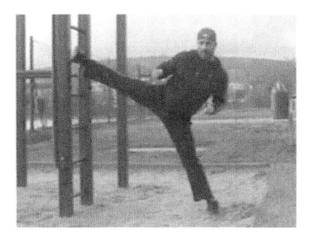

**Hip Flexor Stretch**

Keep your hips facing forward. Feel the stretch in hip flexor. Increase the stretch every 10 seconds. Keep the muscle relaxed. Help it by pushing forward with your arms. After 30 – 40 seconds change legs. Repeat 2 to 3 times for each leg – do 6 sets in total.

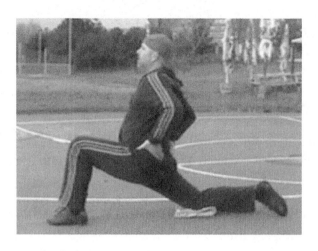

## Elevated Hamstring Stretch

Raise your leg on the wall bar and feel the stretch in your hamstring.

Increase the stretch every 10 seconds without consciously tensing the hamstring. Keep it relaxed. After 30 – 40 seconds change legs. Repeat 2 to 3 times for each leg.

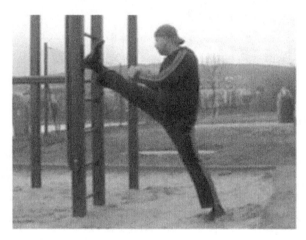

## FLEXIBILITY MAINTENANCE ROUTINE

Congratulations! You've gone through the full 4-week hyperbolic stretching program. It was tough to develop your maximum flexibility and strength, but it wasn't impossible! From now on, things will get much easier, because it is not difficult to maintain your currently flexibility level compared to developing it.

So, what is the secret of flexibility maintenance? First, you don't need to perform the strength training anymore. The only thing you will need to do twice a week is the fourth-week routine mentioned before.

Second, one set of about one minute of sitting in your splits and contracting your muscles in a 5 seconds isometric tension followed by 5 seconds relaxation is all you need to do to keep your maximum flexibility level and your full pelvic floor strength.

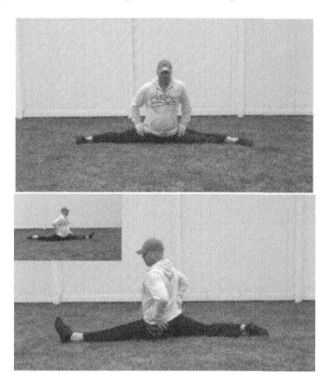

You will save a lot of time that you can invest into stretching other muscles of your body, such as calves, front thighs, glutes, lower and upper back.

With your hip flexors, hamstrings and adductors already flexible, stretching of other muscles will be much easier and quicker. For this purpose, you can use my Full Body Stretching routine that is included in this program in another manual.

## COMPLETE HYPERBOLIC ROUTINE SAMPLE

(Print this page and hang it on the wall at home or in the gym)

### Warm-up session (10 to 15 minutes)

• Joint rotations

• Any aerobic activity to pump blood into your muscles (5 minutes)

• Light warm up stretching

### Your main training session

• Yoga, dancing, martial arts, MMA, weightlifting etc.

• If increasing your flexibility is your only aim, skip this and move to another step

### Flexibility-specific strength training

• Adductor flies – 2 sets of 30 reps till or 1 set of 50+ until muscle burn

• Hamstring curls – 2 sets of 30 or 1 set of 50+ until muscle burn

### Hyperbolic Stretching

• Elevated adductor stretching - 4 sets with 30 sec. rest between sets

• Hip Flexor Stretch – 3 sets on each side with 15 seconds rest

- Elevated hamstring stretching – 3 sets on each side, 15 seconds rest

**Test which of these two stretching protocols suits you best**

**Protocol 1**: Consciously tense your already stretched muscles for 5 seconds applying about 30-40% of maximal tension. Relax for about 3 seconds and increase the stretch. Tense the muscles again for 5 seconds, now with 50% - 60% of your maximal tension. Again, release the tension for 3 seconds and try to increase the stretch. Repeat again, now with maximal tension for 5 seconds, relax and increase the stretch. Now tense again and hold the stretch for at least 12 – 15 seconds. Your set is now over. Change legs and repeat the set. Rest about 60 seconds. Repeat the three times for each leg.

**Protocol 2**: Consciously tense your already stretched muscle for 12-15 seconds applying 30% to 40% of maximal tension. Relax and increase the stretch. Repeat the 12-15 second tension two more times with 50% - 60% of your maximum and then again with 100% of your maximum. Your set is now over. Change legs and repeat the set. Rest about 60 seconds. Repeat the three times for each leg.

## SIMPLIFIED SET FOR PELVIC STRENGTH

(Print this out and hang it on the wall) If you only focus on pelvic strength do this simplified routine.

### Warm-up session (10 to 15 minutes)

Joint rotations, followed by any aerobic activity to pump blood into your muscles (5

minutes), Light Warm Up Stretching using the exercises below. Use the stretching protocol from page 55 and 56.

### Flexibility-specific strength training

•        Adductor flies – 2 sets of 30 reps till or 1 set of 50+ until muscle burn

•        Hamstring curls – 2 sets of 30 or 1 set of 50+ until muscle burn

### Hyperbolic Stretching Simplified

•        Butterfly stretch - 4 sets with 30 sec. rest between sets

•        Hip Flexor Stretch – do 3 sets on each side with 15 seconds rest

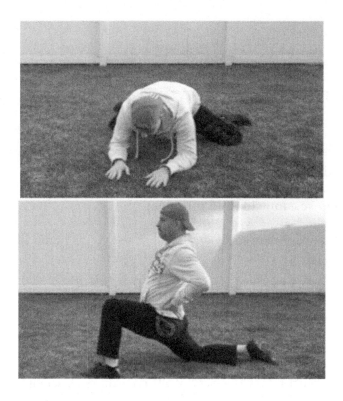

**"Squeeze your muscles as much as you can to strengthen the pelvic floor muscles!"**

**Recommended Stretching Protocol:** Consciously tense your already stretched muscle for 12-15 seconds applying 30% to 40% of maximal tension. Relax and increase the stretch. Repeat the 12-15 second tension two more times with 50% - 60% of your maximum and then again with 100% of your maximum. Your set is now over. Change legs and repeat the set. Rest about 60 seconds. Repeat the three times for each leg.

## MUSCLE SAFETY AND RECOVERY

In every sports manual, safety precautions and recovery techniques need to be addressed. I have already mentioned most of them in previous chapters however muscle recovery was not addressed yet.

Just as in strength training, muscle or hip soreness may happen in stretching especially if you overstretch by accident.

Once this happens, you won't feel like to stretch for few days. The best cure for overstretching and soreness is rest. Additionally, you may take one pill of aspirin before you go to bed.

This will help reduce muscle or hip inflammation and reduce muscle temperature.

Another great thing to implement is to walk up on stairs or do low resistance squats in full range of motion. This will help you recover faster.

If you were stretching slowly, you don't need to be afraid that your muscles or tendons experienced some high-level damage. Your muscles and tendons are very strong and can withstand a lot of force.

Real damage to muscles and tendons only happens by fast unnatural movements – usually in your main training session when you do kicks or some advanced dancing moves.

You should exercise caution though and always be gentle to your body and muscles.

# CONCLUSION

Congratulations if you've made it this far!

If you've gone through the entire 4 week stretching session, you should be able to:

• Do all splits even without warm-up

• Your pelvic muscle strength should be highly developed

• Your glutes are much tighter than ever before

• Your sexual endurance and pleasure should be at its highest peak

• Your erection improved and the ability to have more orgasms should be now completely possible!

You may want to give it all a try!

However, I highly advise that to keep your current condition, you should do the maintenance routine for at least 2 to 3 days per week!

Since the maintenance routine is very short, consider implementing the Full Body Stretching Routine explain in the accompanying book that will help you improve your overall body flexibility even faster!

There is no more tension involved as you will see when you go through the short manual....and it's fun!

I wish you all the best of health and success in your chosen sport discipline! Alex Larsson

# FULL BODY FLEXIBILITY

Despite the fastest way to gain full flexibility is by using hyperbolic and static active stretching protocols, there is yet another type of stretching protocol that deserves your attention.

It is the relaxation stretching protocol that many of you already know from your yoga, dancing or martial arts training. Relaxed stretching is very slow, but very safe way to achieve your full flexibility potential without much muscular effort.

You should implement it into your exercise program, especially after you have gone through the 4-week Hyperbolic Stretching routine and achieved your full lower body flexibility.

There are no tensions involved in this stretching protocol and most of the exercises I am going show you are done performed by sitting or lying on the floor.

If you've searched for the best relaxed stretching exercises, I can honestly tell you that this simple routine covers all your major and smaller muscle groups that needs to be stretched in your lower and upper body.

These exercises are simple to perform. If you are complete newbie to stretching however, I do recommend you to first go through the hyperbolic stretching routine that will help you stretch your thigh muscles first.

Flexible thighs will enable you to use my relaxed stretching routine with no effort as you will be able to assume any position that I am about to share with you.

Another benefit of this routine is that you can use it in your warm-up session, after you went through your joint rotations and at least 5 minutes of aerobic workout of your own choice that have prepared your bodily systems for strenuous activity or your main training session.

So, before you jump into your main training, use the following Full Body Stretching Routine to get your muscles ready to rock and kick! In fact, you can use this stretching routine in your warm up as well as at the end of your training session as a cool-down.

## FULL-BODY RELAXED STRETCHING ROUTINE

Relaxed stretching doesn't cause muscle fatigue. You can perform the routine when your muscles are tired, plus it helps muscle recovery. Relaxed stretching is great as a warm-up or as post workout relaxation. Pay attention to breathing. Assume your stretching position and breathe slowly. Try to increase the stretch by each exhalation.

### Exercise 1 – Standing Stretch

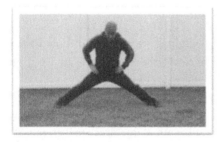 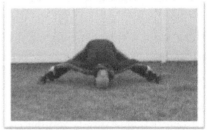

This is an overall upper torso and lower body stretch. It is slightly demanding on muscle strength, balance and stability and will help you warm up your muscles. Make sure you are on a non-slippery surface. Spread your legs and grab your ankles with both hands.

Try touch the floor with your forehead. Hold for 10 seconds.

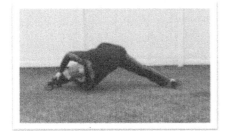 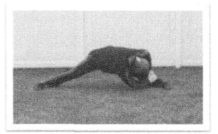

Now, shift your body to right leg and try to touch the floor with your elbow. Hold for 10 seconds and shift to the other leg. Then, shift back toward the center. Do 3 sets in total.

## Exercise 2 – The Piriformis Stretch

You probably know this exercise. It is very beneficial for relieving sciatica, lower back and hip pain. We are going to slightly adjusted version to further relax hips and glutes.

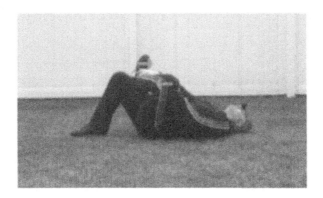

Lay down on your back with both legs bent and feet flat on the ground. Bring your left foot over and place your left ankle over your right thing. Your left knee should face toward your left side. Now, place your right hand on your right ankle and steadily pull it toward your head. At the same time, push with your left knee away from you with your left palm. Do this for 10 to 15 seconds.

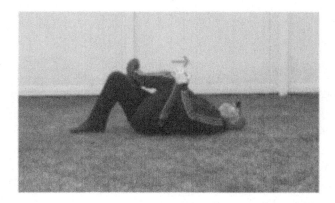

Now, reverse the process. Interlock fingers of both hands behind your left knee and pull toward your right shoulder for 10 to 15 seconds. Then pull that knee away from you again, as seen in the first image. Then pull the knee back to you again. Do total of 2 to 3 sets and then change legs.


**Exercise 3 – Head to Toe Stretch**

This simple exercise targets your hamstrings, calves and lower back muscles.

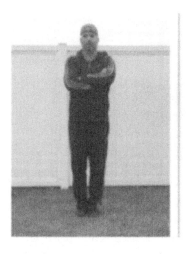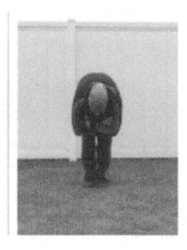

Interlock your arms, straighten your knees and bend over toward your knees. Let the weight of your upper body increase your stretch with every exhalation. Stay in this position for at least 20 seconds. Repeat 2 to 3 times with 5 seconds rest between sets.

**Exercise 4 – Toe Flex**

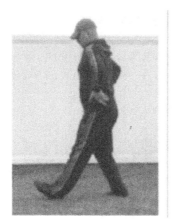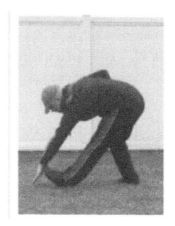

Put one foot in front of you and flex the toe. Transfer your body weight on the slightly bent rear leg. Bend over and try to touch your toe with your left hand. Increase the stretch with every exhalation. Use your extended arm as a measurement tool for every incremental stretch you gain in the exercise. Hold for 10 seconds. Do 2 sets for each leg.

**Exercise 5 – Drop Stance Stretch**

This exercise targets hip flexors, lower back muscles, hamstrings, calves and adductors.

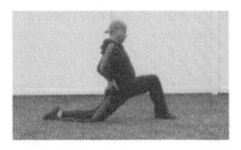

Drop into the hip flexor stretch and push your pelvis forward to stretch your psoas muscle (hip flexor) as much as you can. Hold for 15 seconds.

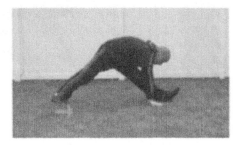

Straighten both legs and bend forward as much as you can. My rear foot is points forward as much as possible for additional stretch of my calf muscle. Hold 15 seconds.

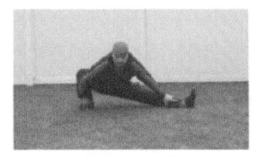

Sit down on your right leg with knee out a 45-degree angle. Hold your right ankle with your right palm and pull your right knee to the back with your right elbow. Hold for 15 seconds. Do 2 sets for each side.

**Exercise 6 – Straddle Split Stretch**

This exercise targets adductors, upper, lower back muscles, hamstrings and adductors.

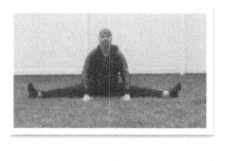 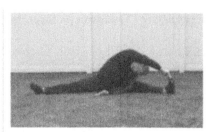

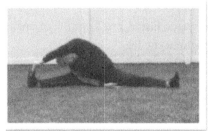 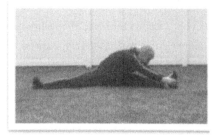

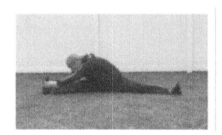 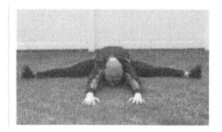

Spread your legs as far apart as you can. Raise your arms overhead and bend sideways, trying to reach your toe with your hand. If you are not able to reach it, you can use slow and mild bouncing movement to increase the stretch. Hold for 10 seconds, then bend over to the other leg. After another ten seconds shift your body on the other side but this time, your torso should face your thing. Reach for your toe and hold 15 seconds.

Move to the other leg. Come back to the center and bring your chest toward the floor. Stretch your arms out in front. Hold for 15 seconds. Repeat the entire cycle 3 times.

### Exercise 6 – Quadriceps Stretch

Hold on to a wall or chair. Grab ankle of your right leg and pull your heel toward your buttocks.

Keep your torso upright.

Hold for 20 seconds, feeling and increasing the stretch of your quadriceps. Repeat 3 times for each leg.

If you want to increase flexibility of your quads faster, press with your ankle against your arm, as if you wanted to straighten the leg.

Use one of the two standard hyperbolic stretching protocols, i.e. tense for 5 seconds – relax – increase the stretch – tense again etc.

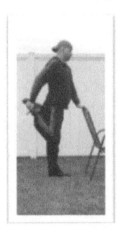

### Exercise 6 – Abdominal Stretch

This exercise targets your abdominal muscles and your hip flexors. It is the safest exercise for abdominal muscles I know.

If your core muscles and abdomen isn't conditioned, avoid doing bridges as they tend to develop excessive tension-stretch that can result in abdominal hernia.

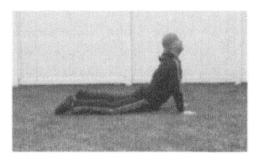

Lay flat on the floor and spread your legs slightly apart. Raise your upper body off the floor but keep your pelvis firmly in the floor. Stay in this position for 10 to 20 seconds. Feel the stretch in your abdomen.

Try to increase the stretch every 5 seconds. Repeat 3 to 4 times.

## DYNAMIC WARM-UP

Although I am personally not convinced, scientific research has shown that dynamic stretching that involves different movements of limbs is the best way to prepare your body for your main training session or competition.

I personally believe that static stretches followed by dynamic movements that resemble the actual movents of your sports discipline done in a progressive fashion – first slowly and low and then quickly and higher works better. At least for the sports I am interested in – which is martial arts and MMA.

However, you may want to follow scientific recommendations. In fact, for some sports (such as golf) plain dynamic stretching can be indeed much better than the static- dynamic warm-ups I personally prefer.

Here's the reasoning and the basic routine you can follow to warm-up your body using dynamic stretching.

Science has moved on. Researchers now believe that some of the more entrenched elements of many athletes' warm-up regimens are not only a waste of time but actually bad for you. The old presumption that holding a stretch for 20 to 30 seconds — known as static stretching — primes muscles for a workout is dead wrong. It actually weakens them, which is true as I explained on my website and in my main book.

In a recent study conducted at the University of Nevada, Las Vegas, athletes generated less force from their leg muscles after static stretching than they did after not stretching at all. Other studies have found that this stretching decreases muscle strength by as much as 30 percent. Also, stretching one leg's muscles can reduce strength in the other leg as well, probably because the central nervous system rebels against the movements.

There is a neuromuscular inhibitory response to static stretching. The straining muscle becomes less responsive and stays weakened for up to 30 minutes after stretching, which is not how an athlete wants to begin a workout. The right warm-up should do two things: loosen muscles and tendons to increase the range of motion of various joints, and literally warm up the body. When you're at rest, there's less blood flow to muscles and tendons, and they stiffen. You need to make tissues and tendons compliant before beginning exercise.

A well-designed warm-up starts by increasing body heat and blood flow. Warm muscles and dilated blood vessels pull oxygen from the bloodstream more efficiently and use stored muscle fuel more effectively. They also withstand loads better.

One significant if gruesome study found that the leg-muscle tissue of laboratory rabbits could be stretched farther before ripping if it had been electronically stimulated — that is, warmed up. To raise the body's temperature, a warm-up must begin with aerobic activity, usually light jogging. Most coaches and athletes have known this for years.

That's why tennis players run around the court four or five times before a match and marathoners stride in front of the starting line. But many athletes do this portion of their warm-up too intensely or too early. A 2002 study of collegiate volleyball players found that those who'd warmed up and then sat on the bench for 30 minutes had lower

backs that were stiffer than they had been before the warm-up.

And a number of recent studies have demonstrated that an overly vigorous aerobic warm-up simply makes you tired. Most experts advise starting your warm-up jog at about 40 percent of your maximum heart rate (a very easy pace) and progressing to about 60 percent. The aerobic warm-up should take only 5 to 10 minutes, with a 5- minute recovery. (Sprinters require longer warm-ups, because the loads exerted on their muscles are so extreme.) Then it's time for the most important and unorthodox part of a proper warm-up regimen, the Spider-Man and its counterparts.

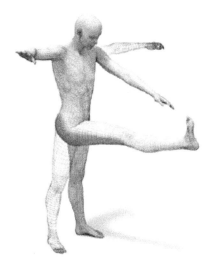

STRAIGHT-LEG MARCH for the hamstrings and gluteus muscles. Kick one leg straight out in front of you, with your toes flexed toward the sky. Reach your opposite arm to the upturned toes. Drop the leg and repeat with the opposite limbs. Continue the sequence for at least six or seven repetitions.

While static stretching is still almost universally practiced among amateur athletes — watch your child's soccer team next weekend — it doesn't improve the muscles' ability to perform with more power, physiologists now agree. You may feel as if you're able to stretch farther after holding a stretch for 30 seconds.

But typically you've increased only your mental tolerance for the discomfort of the stretch. The muscle is actually weaker. Stretching muscles while moving, on the other hand, a technique known as dynamic stretching or dynamic warm-ups, increases power, flexibility and range of motion. Muscles in motion don't experience that insidious inhibitory response. They instead get an excitatory message to perform.

Dynamic stretching is at its most effective when it's relatively sports specific. You need range-of-motion exercises that activate all the joints and connective tissue that will be needed for the task ahead. For runners, an ideal warm-up might include squats, lunges and "form drills" like kicking your buttocks with your heels. Athletes who need to move rapidly in different directions, like soccer, tennis or basketball players, should do dynamic stretches that involve many parts of the body.

"Spider-Man" is a particularly good drill: drop onto all fours and crawl the width of the court, as if you were climbing a wall. Even golfers, notoriously nonchalant about warming up (a recent survey of 304 recreational golfers found that two-thirds seldom or never bother), would benefit from exerting themselves a bit before teeing off.

In one 2004 study, golfers who did dynamic warm-up exercises and practice swings increased their clubhead speed and were projected to have dropped their handicaps by seven strokes over seven weeks. Controversy remains about the extent to which dynamic warm-ups prevent injury. But studies have been increasingly clear that static stretching alone before exercise does little or nothing to help. The largest study has been done on military recruits; results showed that an almost equal number of subjects developed lower-limb injuries (shin splints, stress fractures, etc.), regardless of whether they had performed static stretches before training sessions.

A major study published earlier this year by the Centers for Disease Control, on the other hand, found that knee injuries were cut nearly in half among female collegiate soccer players who followed a warm-up program that included both dynamic warm-up exercises and static stretching. And in golf, those who warm up are nine times less likely to be injured.

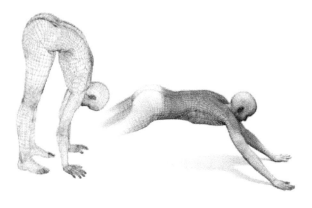

HANDWALKS (for the shoulders, core muscles and hamstrings) Stand straight, with your legs together. Bend over until both hands are flat on the ground. "Walk" your hands forward until your back is almost extended. Keeping your legs straight, inch your feet toward your hands, then walk your hands forward again. Repeat five or six times.

You're Getting Warmer: The Best Dynamic Stretches

These exercises are good for many athletes, even golfers. Do them immediately after your aerobic warm-up and as soon as possible before your workout.

STRAIGHT-LEG MARCH (for the hamstrings and gluteus muscles)

Kick one leg straight out in front of you, with your toes flexed toward the sky. Reach your opposite arm to the upturned toes. Drop the leg and repeat with the opposite limbs. Continue the sequence for at least six or seven repetitions.

SCORPION (for the lower back, hip flexors and gluteus muscles)

Lie on your stomach, with your arms outstretched and your feet flexed so that only your toes are touching the ground. Kick your right foot toward your left arm, then kick your left foot toward your right arm. Since this is an advanced exercise, begin slowly, and repeat up to 12 times.

HANDWALKS (for the shoulders, core muscles, and hamstrings)

Stand straight, with your legs together. Bend over until both hands are flat on the ground. "Walk" with your hands forward until your back is almost extended. Keeping your legs straight, inch your feet toward your hands, then walk your hands forward again. Repeat five or six times.

# MIND POWER UNLEASHED

I sincerely invite you to take part on a miraculous journey to your own Desire Fulfillment. These extremely powerful result-oriented techniques address over 130 difficult life conditions and approach these issues from perspectives of psychology, spirituality and personal development.

All mind manifestation systems recognized that the difference between poverty and wealth or between sickness and health lies in depths of human mind. The only barrier that stands in the way of your desire manifestation are the thoughts you think and the words you speak. Over years, your thoughts and words molded false beliefs that have been unconsciously rooted and held in the back of your mind. To bring abundance into life or achieve anything you want in life, you need to first organize content of your deeper (unconscious) mind first.

The rest will follow.

Mind reprogramming has been part of humanity for centuries and after rigorous studies and testing, I am sure that modern science of psychology often overlaps with the ancient secrets. Method you are going to discover on the following pages has been successfully tested on top athletes, top managers and entrepreneurs. Keep an open mind and see if you can some of it in your own life.

You are free to adjust these techniques according to your own personal beliefs and world views. Take this manual as a template out of which your own deeply intimate system of mind power will be created. In this manual we will go deeply within human desires and far back in time and space.

Remember the saying: "If you want to create an apple pie from the scratch,

you must first create the universe."

Alex Larsson

## HEALING STATEMENTS

If you've ever heard about affirmations, you will quickly get a grasp of what the Healing Statement Method is all about. Healing Statements (also known as "Magnets") are highly structured sets of sentences that have been proven to work much more effectively than short affirmations you may have learned from other sources.

Healing Statements are basically 10 to 15 sentence-long 'declarations' or 'sets of arguments' designed to effectively and quickly reprogram your Subconscious Mind (confirmed by modern psychology to produce your daily habits and attract everyday experiences) in such a way that your mind will start working on manifesting your desires almost immediately.

Each sentence in a single Healing Statement (Magnet) builds upon previous one and all sentences together act similarly as a motivational speech that sports coaches give to their teams before an important sports match.

Such a coherent and intelligently structured string of arguments quickly removes old false beliefs from subconscious mind, planting new productive 'belief seeds' that draw abundance of wealth, health and love into your life, reversing any of the 130+ negative life issues listed in this workbook.

Unlike other manifestation or law of attraction systems that rely on simple affirmations or visualization techniques that at best help you change your daily habits, Healing Statements (Magnets) have the capability to change your life circumstances completely, creating a whole new life-reality that is in perfect conformity with your Will.

Active Ingredients in Healing Statements

In their essence, Healing Statements contain two active manifestation ingredients: The psychological power of reasoning and the psychological element of so-called 'third party' of Collective Unconscious, rediscovered by the famous psychoanalyst Carl Gustav Jung and further elaborated by Roberto Assagioli and Lionell Corbett.

Currently, the term Collective Unconscious is often being rephrased as 'objective psyche' or as 'autonomous psyche' among many modern neuroscientists and manifestation experts who study and test this remarkable phenomenon.

These two elements make new things manifest in your life fast. I will explain more in coming chapters but let me elaborate on this a little right now.

In your Healing Statement, you'll be mentioning a "third-party" that I like to call the 'Infinite Mind' or 'Endless Mind' throughout this manual. The Endless Mind should be understood to represent the Collective Unconscious or Objective Mind that is not part of your own (subjective) mind.

Using this 'third-party element' represented by something infinitely powerful, all knowing, omnipresent and incomprehensible to human mind helps reprogram content of your subconscious mind faster.

To show you how a Healing Statement (Magnet) works and how it gains unusual amount of power from "supporting arguments" and the "third-party", let me compare it to a simple affirmation.

If you're using simple affirmation, such as 'Every day, I am feeling better and better" despite in your real life you are feeling worse and worse, you are basically lying to yourself. Your subconscious mind will reject the new thought contained in the affirmation.

You are basically telling yourself something that doesn't fit the script upon which your body and subconscious mind currently operate. Trust me, subconscious mind does not like to accept new conflicting thoughts into its realm just as you don't like to be disturbed when you're focusing on some task at hand.

In fact, your subconscious mind rejects new thoughts from its system on daily basis. It works against new thoughts and beliefs simply because these new thoughts don't resonate with what the deeper mind was told to do for years.

Yes, subconscious mind does record all new thoughts and impulses from the environment around you, but your subconscious mind does not act on impulses that do not fit its framework of operation.

These impulses are simply being edited and censored, marked as unimportant and then stored into an 'archive folder' within your subconscious mind. Therefore, every single day you may be missing on hundreds of important inceptions, ideas and opportunities that are just a breath away from you – those that could improve your life for the better.

Deeper (subconscious) mind works according old patterns, totally independently of your conscious mind and Will. And since most people do not have "good relationship" with their subconscious minds, they fail changing their habits and lives simply because they are not acting upon impulses that may have the capability to open new pathways to life they've always wanted to live.

People are often unknowingly being forced to live their entire lives using the same old patterns. There is simply nothing new or positive happening in their lives thanks to the 'editor' and 'censorship' on their subconscious level. In addition, using some simple affirmation that isn't part of your reality now may put yourself into huge stress because you are basically pushing yourself into believing something that isn't yet true.

By stating 'I am getting richer and richer' you are casting a huge chunk of responsibility upon your own psyche, forcing it to deliver something you have absolutely no idea how. This is the reason why, upon years of testing, the manifestation experts introduced the 'third-party' into Healing Statements.

You simply transfer responsibility for desire manifestation to a 'third-party' that 'will take care of the whole thing.'

To make your subconscious mind accept new thoughts and work toward a newly set objective (i.e. feeling better and better, acquire wealth, reverse illness), you need to back yourself up by an authority of the Endless Mind as the source of unknown infinite power behind you.

**Summary:**

Healing Statements represent highly intelligent and structured approach to creating the so-called 'declaration' formulas that work quickly and more effectively than classic affirmations

You will first align your mind with positive attitude by acknowledging Unity with the so-called 'third party.' This will help you quickly reprogram your Subconscious Mind and replace old false beliefs with correct thoughts.

These statements can be effectively used by anyone, in their native language. You can replace the word Endless Mind with the term 'Collective Unconscious' so often elaborated on in highly regarded studies on psychology, particularly in teachings of the famous Carl Gustav Jung and his colleague Roberto Assagioli.

**THERE'S POWER WITHIN YOU**

After successful surgery, a patient comes up to his surgeon to thank him. Surgeon replies: "Don't thank me. It was the invisible Power that did the healing. My task was only to prepare all necessary conditions for the Power of Nature to heal your wounds."

Power of Abundance is the same power that heals and grows everything

new in people's lives, in nature and in the Universe.

We can't see or measure this Power, but we can witness its effects everywhere...

Somewhere back in the hills, there are huge lakes held back by giant dams. Natural path of water from of those lakes is diverted, so it flows over large turbines that produce electricity.

You may liken an individual to an electric light bulb. Light manifests through it, yet it is not produced by it.

Conducted through high tension wires, electricity generated by turbines passes through transformers which then pass it through network of wires down to a household located in nearby city.

Thus, the electricity is led from its power source into the tiniest wire of all, the wire within the bulb. This tiny bulb is an outlet of the Powerful Source located far away in hills.

And so are we, locked far away from our very own Source, trapped in this body of flesh in Material Universe, also called World of Action, a plane of coarse matter...while The Source is hidden in the subtlest sphere far beyond our ability to see It.

In fact, this makes perfect sense because if we were in constant visual presence of the Source, we would not be able to make any decisions on our own. Our free will would be non-existent because we would be living in a never-ending awe of God's greatness.

Some call this Source Power of Abundance, God, Yah, Jehovah, Allah, Brahman or Buddha. Others call it Quantum Field, Subtle Energy, Chi, Qi, Ki or Higher Intelligence but meaning is still the same. Essentially, the Source and the Power are the very same thing since everything that exists is in fact, a one single Unified Whole.

But to study it, ancient masters as well as modern scientists had to divide this Whole into parts, because if everything in Universe was considered as One Single Whole, then there would be nothing to study.

We are talking about the same Power every time, regardless of what belief system we follow. Yet, this power has two extreme sides. On one side, it is characterized by anabolic qualities that create everything new and positive in Universe and on the other side, it is responsible for everything destructive and restrictive.

This program is not about motivation. With all honesty and respect, motivation is not as effective as many people think. Motivation comes and goes while the Power of Abundance grows within you and stays there forever.

As you unblock your own Subconscious Mind and the Power of Abundance starts flowing down to your body and life, you will quickly realize that this Power is going to:

•       serve you the right situations, ideas and opportunities that you've asked for and then…

•       it will drive you to effortlessly achieve your desires

You will physically feel this Power of Abundance within your own body and mind. This is the difference between being simply motivated and being driven by the Power of Abundance.

If we look deeply into old spiritual systems and mainstream religions, we see tiny connections that indicate they all come from one single source – one 'master system' that was long forgotten.

For example, consider the Father of Hebrew nation and his wife's name, Abraham and Sarah – you may notice Hinduism's highest intelligences to be curiously called Brahma and Saraswati, indicating linguistic resemblance with the Hebrew biblical figures.

Same goes for other religions, such as Islam's Allah who has the same root 'Al' in his name as the Jewish El or Elohim, being one of the God's Names revealed in the Old Testament. In addition, if you read Koran, you will find several instances where it tells stories about Jesus.

## LEVELS OF HUMAN MIND

Structure of human mind can be approached from many perspectives, be it scientific or spiritual, so please consider this material as purely introductory.

My effort here is to present you a model that you can apply to your practical manifestation work.

Everything discussed below is in line with teachings of the Kabbalah and the psychology of C. G. Jung, specifically the work of his student and colleague Roberto Assagioli.

I am 100% convinced that these two gentlemen built their knowledge of human mind and soul using ancient sources as there are way too many similarities with the ancient views on human mind.

Here are the four basic levels of human mind and soul (for purpose of this program, we can use these two terms interchangeably):

1.      Superconscious Mind/Soul – the gateway and entrance of inspiration, Divine Will (according to old sages) and new ideas into your conscious awareness – typically illustrated in ancient manuscripts as a round sphere above human head.

2.      Conscious Mind/Soul - Dwelling place of your Ego – Thoughts starting with: I am, I decide, I choose – associated with a sphere positioned on human head (or forehead)

3.      Higher Subconscious Mind/Soul – Trigger of emotions and love – ascribed to the heart level

4.      Middle Subconscious/Unconscious Mind/Soul – Storage of habits and memory, this is your manifestation loom or automatic servant that does not judge its content, stores all content from Conscious Mind, is responsible for automatic bodily functions such as digestion, breathing, heartbeat, metabolism etc. – ascribed to solar plexus or more specifically to liver - the manifestation loom that creates your reality

…including…

Lower Subconscious Mind/Soul – source of survival instincts, fight or flight syndrome, regenerative functions and sexual urges, rough force – associated with genital area.

In this course, you will primarily work with your Conscious Mind and

Middle Subconscious Mind. I will soon explain why.

But first, let me add one more spiritual view on human mind and how it extends beyond the point of your brain.

Your Whole Body Equals Your Mind

Though this may sound contradictory, ancient masters claimed that every cell of your physical body is also part of your mind and soul. From a different view point, this is perfectly in line with current scientific opinion that human thoughts and emotions affect one's physical health.

In fact, many scientists now believe that every cell in your body is a miniature of your mind. All the cells in your body are capable accepting thoughts at their level of operation directly from your Conscious and Subconscious (Deeper) Mind, acting accordingly. This means, that if your subconscious mind is full of negative and destructive thoughts and habits, cells in your body also exhibit destructive and negative patterns of operations which lead to various illnesses and health issues.

Your Environment, People and Events in Your Life

Spiritual masters also believed that just as God's physical body is our physical Universe, our mind is extended into the environment we live in. Starting from aura encompassing your physical body, up to your work, home, friends, family, colleagues, daily situations etc. - this all is also considered part of your body, mind and soul. Your body and mind is the center of yourself, the environment and the people you meet is your circumference, so to speak.

Recall how many times have you asked your friends if they can remind you of some past event? You have used their minds as yours. How many times have you asked other people to do something for you? You used them as your own limbs for some purpose. This again gives sense to the above initial statement.

Lastly, there is one part of mind that modern psychology calls Collective Unconscious (C. G. Jung). According to Jung, Collective Unconscious refers to external structures of subconscious mind that are shared among beings of the same species.

Jung further states that this collective unconscious is populated by instincts and archetypes containing universal symbols such as Wise Old Man, Great Mother, the Shadow, the Tower, Water, Tree of Life and more.

In spiritual circles, this collective mind is called Mind of The Infinite, Endless Mind (elsewhere: Akashic Records) and it is said that to contain all past experiences of the entire human race.

As such, the Endless Mind permeates all worlds bearing qualities of the Creator – i.e. Omnipotence, Omnipresence and Omniscience.

It is your Subconscious Mind that is tightly bound to the Endless Mind and you will be using this relationship to send out conscious commands through your Subconscious Mind directly into the Stream of the Endless Mind, expecting it to come back with solutions to your requests.

You may have noticed that all divisions of your mind I had mentioned, including the external Collective Unconscious literally encompass whole universe. In fact, there is only one Mind/Soul in existence, portion of which is incarnated in your body. The rest is everywhere.

## HOW YOUR MIND WORKS

"By thinking and acting the same way every time, you will be getting the

same results, all the time. Get out of your own way."

For the sake of simplicity, let us consider that you only have two parts of Mind, each having different functions.

Your Conscious [Surface] Mind is one that thinks and decides.

Conscious Mind constantly analyzes everything and then thinks, "I decide to" or "I choose to". It is that part of your Mind that you use when you are dialing phone number or when you are learning to play piano.

Conscious Mind needs to 'think' every number you're about to dial into your cellphone. However, once you learn the phone number or learn to play piano 'by heart', all had already been stored within your Subconscious Mind and your Conscious Mind is that information out of that storage space.

Your Subconscious Mind* stores all your experiences and beliefs including those that were wired into it from your ancestors. This is the reason why when you're dialing that number again, you're not really 'thinking about it'. Your Subconscious Mind does that job for you.

Conscious Mind is on a Higher Level [it has the decision Power] than Subconscious Mind. Your Conscious Mind doesn't have any storage space and therefore it is not bound by experiences from your past nor does it worry about future (because all worries about future come from past experiences).

When Conscious Mind is active, it lives in Presence - just as the un-manifested God lives outside Time, Space and Events without the past or future.

Everything that you consciously think of happens at your Conscious Level only for a tiny little [present] moment and then it fades away or gets stored within your Subconscious Mind.

Subconscious Mind on the other hand, is the real creator of your everyday reality. It is that creative and productive part of our mind that is always looking for impulse or commands from your Conscious Mind.

It takes any thought from Conscious Mind and makes it a reality. Neither does it judge whether an input is good or bad. This part of your Mind is completely automatic and obeys all thoughts, ideas or commands from Conscious Mind.

Subconscious Mind does not have any freedom of choice or any decision power. It accepts any thought produced by the Conscious Mind and acts just like earth, accepting any seed. Unfortunately, Subconscious Mind is habitual.

It works primarily according to commands that you have wired into it repeatedly or with significant (positive or negative) emotional impulse in the past.

Main goal of this program is to provide you with ready-made tools that will help you effortlessly and quickly reprogram your Deeper Mind's old content, regardless of how dominant that content currently is. Since the Subconscious Mind is a reliable agent, we are now aware that changing your thought feed is going to force your Deeper Mind to manifest a whole new reality.

Let us summarize why merely thinking about your desire can't bring you any results...

## WHY PRAYERS ARE NOT HEARD

We all pray and have desires. Yet our prayers go by unheard. However, the Universe does not give us desires because he wants to torture us or block their fulfilment. He gives them to us because he wants them to be fulfilled. It is us who stand in our own way. More precisely, our old beliefs. There are two possible reasons why we are not getting what we want.

### Inhibiting Beliefs

Life is driven by Principles and Laws. Let us briefly look at the most prominent one - the Law of Cause and Effect.

If you plant an onion, you can't expect that a rose grows up from the onion seed. This also applies to beliefs and doubts you hold in your Deeper Mind. You need to root these out and replace them with new, correct thoughts to experience new results that will be in conformity with your will.

In other words, these old inhibiting beliefs represent blocks at the subconscious level. This blocks partially inhibit free flow of the abundant energy that already IS passing through your body and out into your life in certain amount.

This is where Healing Statements come in. This intelligent way of short structured commands can wipe off all your limiting beliefs almost immediately, replacing them with correct and positive thoughts, forcing your Subconscious Mind to work on your behalf automatically.

But as I said in the promotional video, that's not all. Despite the Healing

Statements work effectively on their own, my method goes far beyond that.

If you want to increase the power of Healing Statements, you can add the Names of Power into your manifestation session and experience faster results.

## HOW DESIRE COMES TO YOU

This is an important part missed by many practitioners. As you will soon see, you first exercise will be to get a better picture about your desire.

This little practice will help you pin down your desire into its final material form.

However, you need to let your Deeper Mind decide how the outcome eventually manifests. In the actual Healing Statement, you want to present your request in more general terms.

Being part of the Endless Mind, your Subconscious Mind knows better and selects the best way to manifest your desire.

When the energy of abundance starts flowing down to your Subconscious Mind, it will pick up all the information about the desire you've written down on paper.

Deeper Mind then sends this information out to the Endless (Collective) Mind that will bring about the result.

### Unlimited Resources of Subconscious Mind

In previous chapters, we have discussed the relationship between Conscious and Subconscious Mind and how you can influence one with the other to achieve a positive change in your life.

In this chapter, we will look at how the Subconscious Mind relates to the Endless Mind and how it can use its unlimited resources to bring about the change within your life almost instantly.

Subconscious Mind is often termed as the Manifestation Loom and since it has direct connection to the Endless Mind, it has access to all experiences of the entire human race.

It remembers all stories of how a wealth or success was built in every corner of this Planet at any given moment of time. It knows everything about healing of any disease that ever took place and even how every love or relationship started or was restored.

The Endless Mind has all the knowledge and all the Power to achieve anything. You just need to feed your Subconscious Mind with proper commands, so it can reach out to the Endless Mind and manifest the results you want.

The Endless Mind doesn't live in the past or future. It lives in Presence that contains all past events and all possibilities of future. Likewise, the Endless Mind doesn't know any distance because it is part of everything. It is Omnipresent.

This means there is no time and distance limit on when, where and how your desire manifests.


**Cause and Effect Revisited**

As I mentioned previously, nothing is wasted in the Universe. Every positive or negative thought and deed comes back to you, sooner or later.

The Universe is fair. It never fails to disappoint you. The only one who can disappoint yourself is you – just as I am disappointing myself in that I give wrong instructions to my own Subconscious Mind.

But it's not your fault, because until now you didn't have this knowledge. It took me long time to realize that I was sabotaging my own progress by planting wrong thoughts, beliefs and opinions into myself.

It may be difficult to stop thinking negatively, but this can be learned in steps. First, when negative thought pops up in your mind, observe it but never manifest this thought by expressing it loudly. Just let it fade away from your mind. It only requires to be a little calm and to control your emotions little more.

Avoid negative conversation. If you speak with someone whose mouth is full of negative stories, try to change the subject and if it doesn't work, leave.

Every person 'spreads seeds' every time he or she thinks and speaks. Positive and negative, all thoughts grow silently along each other. It is only a matter of time when you harvest what you had planted.

This means that by right of consciousness you are exactly on the spot where you are meant to be, right now. From now on, plant your thought seeds carefully and wisely. There is no fate, only your planted seeds.

Once you understand this concept, you can start planting new seeds and expect positive changes. When? Remember there is no time or distance limit to the Endless Mind, so expect results very, very fast.


## What Are We Really Healing

The Manifestation Masterkey is all about activating inner process of healing that results in manifestation of your desire. You will use a special Healing Statement with the intent of producing desired change in your mind, body and life that will be in conformity with your will.

But why do I call it a healing? Because Healing is an act of Unification. When you cut yourself the two split sides of your skin need to unify to remove the opening. In fact, all lack of financial resources, every illness, lack of health and love, even hate and envy is perceived as a separation from the abundant energy that grows and maintains everything in the Universe.

In ancient times, all human thoughts that were not directed to the Supreme God were perceived as Evil. Thus, by pointing your thoughts toward the abundance, you are not only healing your body or changing some of your life circumstances.

You are healing your thought process by changing your mind's content.

Once you replace your old false beliefs, external changes will happen automatically. You are healing the cause, not the effect here. Real healing takes place in your Subconscious Mind.

Don't think of money and what you can buy for it. Think of the Universal Principle of Abundance and the money will follow. Prosperity is not primarily money, it is a deep internal state of your mind out of which money grow in one way or the other.

We recognize seven core False Beliefs, that are also known as the Parent Thoughts. These Parent Thoughts are at root of your thinking. Remove the Parent thoughts so they don't give birth the off-springs – those other, smaller false beliefs that you may be holding in the back of your mind.

Change one dominant Parent Thought (Core False Belief) and all the rest of incorrect beliefs are going to fall apart in no time. In fact, changing just one single Core Parent Thought also weakens any other of the seven Core Parent Thoughts within your mind.

So, you only need to select one Healing Statement (Magnet) that removes just one Core Parent Thought and work only with that. You don't need to use any other of the remaining six Healing Statements whatsoever.

A Core False Belief related to lack of financial resources, prosperity and wealth is called The Parent Thought of Vanity, Futility and Overload.

Deep in your mind, you may believe that you're far away from all the wealth and prosperity. You may think that you don't have the necessary knowledge, luck, skills or will to reach the financial freedom you want.

That is of course, not true.

You need to replace this Parent Thought of Vanity, Futility and Overload with what I call a Master Thought – in this case it is the Master Thought of Adequacy and Resourcefulness.

This Correct Thought will make you internally convinced that you have all the power and resources to acquire wealth and financial freedom. This new belief will be released by your Subconscious Mind into Endless Mind that will take care of the rest and manifest the wealth in your life.

Using this very same Master Thought, I built my own wealth with only a

$360 in my pocket. I found a business opportunity when I was shopping in a local discount store. I found a tiny little product and suddenly, I envisioned myself placing an offer of this product on the internet.

I did just that and it proved to be the right thing.

Something inside my own being was driving me to take advantage of this opportunity. I was so convinced about the success that there was nothing that could have stopped me from acting and posting the product offer on-line.

Today, my brand sells over 30 different home products and almost all parts of my daily business operations has been outsourced, leaving me with more time to focus on enjoying my life. Since the Endless Mind knows how every of success and business was built, once you tap into this resource all the money, wealth and prosperity will start to manifest fast.

You already have all the resources at your fingertips – just give it a try.

Theory of False Beliefs states that past ancestors of every person developed certain beliefs about life and these have been stored deeply within each individual Subconscious Mind. Other false beliefs may have molded during our own lives as a result of upbringing or negative situations and event.

People who come from long lineage of poor ancestors who never experienced any significant success tend to have the False Belief of Vanity, Futility and Overload rooted more powerfully than those who come from richer lineages.

Add negative experiences and beliefs you've picked up in your current life and see this Core False Belief increase in strength, further negatively influencing your level of prosperity.

With regards to health, it works the same way. Man does not only think with his brain, he thinks with his whole body. Every cell in your body takes information from your Subconscious Mind and adapts to its content.

Cells in your body are not able to think independently, so they follow commands from your Subconscious Mind. Everything that comes out of your mind becomes a specimen or pattern that every cell in your body follows.

If you often feel irritated, your cells get irritated too. And since every thought constantly looks for an outlet, you may end up being diagnosed with inflammation on your skin or with a stomach ulcer.

Over years, this irritating mindset is going to infuse all cells in your body with irritation. Eventually, you may find yourself exhibiting irritation toward people and life in general. Not to say that this negative thought can cause even more damage to your overall health.

From spiritual perspective, the Universe only thinks perfect thoughts through us. The Universe sees everything as perfect. It is us who adopt different, often negative views on everything, thus blocking the flow of perfect thoughts the Universe wants to think through our minds.

We must let the Universe think its perfect thoughts through us.

Man needs the Infinite Universe (the Endless Mind) for Power and Infinite Universe needs man as an outlet for its power of abundance to manifest.

## HOW DESIRE COMES TO YOU

Do this little exercise prior to your first manifestation session. You only need to do this once for each desire you want to see manifested in your life.

Sit down in a quiet place where you won't be disturbed. With pen and paper in your hands, spend couple of minutes thinking about your desire. This exercise is essential in preparing your Subconscious Mind so that it can take over your desire. IT needs to know what it is you really want and why.

Write following four questions down. Contemplate each question and write down definitive answers on each. Be fully honest to yourself and don't hold back. There is no good or bad answer here. Choose only one objective at a time and write as much as you can next to each question.

Questions for Wealth, Money and Prosperity Manifestation:

1.      How much money, am I asking for exactly?

2.      Why do I need the money?

3.      What will I use the money for and why do I want the money?

4.      What am I willing to sacrifice for manifestation of this desire?

Last question is very important. You don't want to sacrifice too much. But

you need to come up with an answer.

Remember, in the Universe "Nothing is for Free" and this is a Law.

This Law has also been long known in modern physics as the Law of Conservation Energy, defined by Rudolph Clausius in 1850. If you ask for

something you wouldn't normally get in your life, some amount of a subtle energy will have to be exerted to manifestation of your desire.

And that energy will have to be replaced in one way or the other from your own resources. If you define what you are willing to sacrifice before working your manifestation sessions, your total loss will equal to what you were willing to sacrifice

I usually sacrifice some small tangible thing in my possession that I had purchased in my past. It can also be food or a drop of an olive oil.

Recently, a new student asked me: "Alex, why can't I sacrifice let's say poverty?" I answered: You should always sacrifice something that is of value to you.

IF there is an Intelligent Being out there, it may not be fond of receiving a poverty in exchange for favor.

If you are a purist and want to go an extra mile, you can create a small altar in your backyard or in the nearby forest and donate i.e. food leftovers to it, once per week. Another great idea is to recite your Healing Statement right there at the altar or the place where you regularly donate your sacrifice.

So, here are the questions you want to have answered in detail before your first manifestation session.

Questions for Health Manifestation:

1.       What exactly do I want to heal?

2.       Why exactly do I want to get healed?

3.       What will I do when I get healed?

4.       What am I willing to sacrifice for manifestation of this desire? Questions for New Relationship

Manifestation:

1.       What are the criteria for my new partner, what do I expect from him and what can I give him in return?

2.       Why do I want new relationship?

3.       What changes do I expect in my life once I have the new partner in my life?

4.       What am I willing to sacrifice for manifestation of this desire? Questions for Existing Relationship

Restoration:

1.    What do I want to improve in my current relationship?

2.    Why do I want to improve my current relationship?

3.    What changes do I expect in my life when my current relationship improves?

4.    What am I willing to sacrifice for manifestation of this desire?

## PRE-DONE STATEMENTS FOR WEALTH & HEALTH

Income follows consciousness. Jesus once said: "Unto everyone that hath shall be given, but for him that hath not shall be taken away even that which he hath". This one is indeed harsh, but it draws the picture of what he was trying to say – that man's thoughts do have power and that you should cultivate money your consciousness. And that is exactly what the Healing Statements are all about.

In this chapter, you will find seven ready-made Healing Statements. Each one is designed to wipe out one of the seven Core False Beliefs (Parent Thoughts) from your Subconscious Mind, replacing them with Correct Master Thought.

Simply go over each Healing Statement and find the one that best relates to the problem or issue you want to solve.

If you don't find your problem listed below, pick the False Belief #1: Vanity,

Futility and Overload or False Belief #3: Loss and Separation.

If you prefer creating your own Healing Statement, you can take any ready-made statement and adjust the Reasoning Part to better reflect your current situation.

Just be careful not to change other parts of each statement as the other parts are inevitable for full manifestation.

You can rewrite your chosen Healing Statement into your PC text editor or into your smartphone and adjust it right there. You can also write it down on a piece of paper and spend day or two memorizing it. If you find memorization difficult, you can read it loudly from the paper, PC or smartphone once, maximum two times per day.

Ideally you want to recite it once loudly in the morning and then silently in your mind in the evening. Or vice versa.

As I said previously, you can replace the Endless Mind with any word that better reflects your personal beliefs and world view

For maximum effect, please try not to miss any session and stick to it for minimum of 21 days.

These are the universal components of a properly structured Healing Statement:

1.     The Opening Part where you are going to align yourself with the structure of the universe, recognizing its powers: I am the extension of the Endless Mind. Endless Mind never runs away from anything, ever for It is Omnipotent, Omnipresent and All-Knowing. Therefore, what's valid for the Endless Mind is also valid for me and I am completely infused by Its Universal Power.

2.     Reasoning Part – you can adjust this part. Here, you are using arguments to take away all doubts.

3.     The Realization Part where you reconfirm the reasoning part with

following statement: "This is the Truth and it is so."

4.     The Release Part where you acknowledge that your desire was

released into the Endless Mind and the result is fully in the Endless Mind's hands. Here, it is important that you 'release your desire' with absolute confidence in the power of the Endless Mind: I now release this thought into the Endless Mind.

5.      The Rejoicing Part where you thank the Endless Mind with the expectancy of results: I thank the Endless Mind for full manifestation of my desire.

What follows are the seven pre-done Healing Statements. Each replaces one of the core false beliefs with correct thought.

Stick to one Healing Statement for at least 21 days. I have also created small workbooks with the mostly used Healing Statements – I call these 'Magnets' or 'Sample Procedures'. You can find them in your Membership Account.

False Belief #1: Vanity, Futility, Overload: ("I can't get through this")

Income follows consciousness. This false belief is the main inhibitor of wealth, money influx, financial success and prosperity

Correct Thought #1: Adequacy and Resourcefulness ("My power is enough for everything")

Removes: alcoholism, anemia, anxiety, asthma, cerebral hemorrhage, diabetes, envy, enlarged, tired and palpitated heart, hemorrhoids, hernia, high blood pressure, complex of inferiority, insanity, nervous breakdown, overweight, paralysis, prolapsed organs, sadism

Healing Statement:

I am the extension of the Endless Mind. The Endless Mind never runs away from anything, ever, for It is Omnipotent, Omnipresent and All-Knowing.

Therefore, what's valid for the Endless Mind is also valid for me and I am completely infused by this Universal Power.

Any barrier or load is less than I am, because I as mind am superior to it. Since I am an extension the Endless Mind, I can easily carry any load. Great reserves are built into my body and unplumbed depths of power dwell in my mind.

They're so infinite that nothing can come against me. I am fit to face life at any point. I refuse to allow negative thoughts sneak into the citadel of my thinking. They can't enter without my invitation. I refuse them to enter.

This is the Truth and it is so.

I now release this thought into the Endless Mind. I thank the Endless Mind for full manifestation of my desire.

False Belief #2: Delays and Obstructions ("This person or thing blocks me")

This belief stops all your efforts and desires before they manifest. If you have this thought as dominant one, you're probably experiencing nothing but failures in business, at work and in relationships. You also may have a problem with finishing tasks at work or in your life in general.

Correct Thought #2: Resistlessness ("Nothing can stand in the way of resistless flow God/Endless Mind.")

Removes: circulation, cataract, constipation, closing sales, coronary occlusion, deafness, delay in love and marriage, embolism, getting loans, getting a raise, hardening of arteries, promotion in business, sale of property)

**Healing Statement:**

I am the extension of the Endless Mind. The Endless Mind never sees an obstruction, ever, for It is Omnipotent, Omnipresent and All-Knowing. Therefore, what's valid for the Endless Mind is also valid for me and I am completely infused by this Universal Power.

Obstacles I seem to see in the outer world arise within myself, because of false beliefs that I have about myself and about the universe. A barrier to one person is simply a hurdle for another.

I rest in the assurance that what I desire is only the out-thrust of the Endless Mind in me seeking its fullest expression. The Endless Mind sees nothing that wishes to obstruct IT or that would be able to.

I range myself alongside the Endless Mind and fill my own mind with the assurance of the resistless flow of the Infinite Will through me.

False Belief #3: Loss and Separation

People with this dominant thought are often rebelling against authorities and experience many injuries during their life span.

Such a person is always anti-social, accusing others, hates others and fears of being misused. He or she often ends up in hospital or jail.

Correct Thought #3: Inseparable Unity and Oneness ("Nothing is ever lost in the Mind of God")

Removes: Loss of organ function and sanity. Loss of prosperity, job, business, customers or sales. Loss of love, beauty, youth. Loss of loved ones and friends.

**Healing Statement:**

I am the extension of the Endless Mind. The Endless Mind never sees an obstruction, ever, for It is Omnipotent, Omnipresent and All-Knowing. Therefore, what's valid for the Endless Mind is also valid for me and I am completely infused by this Universal Power.

Nothing is ever lost to the Endless Mind. What I call loss is only my inability to see this valued thing now or my inability to know where it is. Principle of conservation of energy and matter tells me that nothing is ever lost in the Universe – it only changes location.

The Subconscious Mind in me already knows where my desired thing is. It also knows where I am. It brings me to it, or it to me. It shows me exactly how to get reunited with that which appears to me as lost.

I do not accept the idea of loss whatsoever in my life. I know that in my life everything is in complete union and I am always at the right place.

False Belief #4: Irritation

This false belief usually manifests as an impatience or irritation toward other people who are either different than us or react and think differently than we do.

Correct Thought #4: Tranquility

Removes: Eczema and all skin irritations, all conditions ending with "itis" that mean inflammation, ulcers, shingles, catarrh, sinus trouble, gall bladder issues, hypersensitiveness to criticism, intolerance of "different" people

Healing Statement:

I am the extension of the Endless Mind. The Endless Mind never sees an obstruction, ever, for It is Omnipotent, Omnipresent and All-Knowing. Therefore, what's valid for the Endless Mind is also valid for me and I am completely infused by this Universal Power.

There is a world within me that is completely free from any kind of

irritation. It's the hidden dwelling place of the Universal Power, where

tranquility reigns supreme.

Nothing can enter this place without my consent. I refuse this place to be disturbed by any type of intruder. My mind is calm in the face of million aggravations. This Power thinks its peace through me.

This is the Truth and it is so.

I now release this thought into the Endless Mind. I thank the Endless Mind for full manifestation of my desire.


False Belief #5: Hostility and Cross-Purposes ("People are against me.")

This false belief comes from your ancestors as a direct result of wars and competition for life and food. People who like to compete in business or sports often have this belief dominant.

Correct Thought #5: No competition ("There are enough resources for everyone")

Removes: Allergies, virus, asthma in children, migraines, fever, bacterial infections, unexplainable hostility of others against you, leukemia, gossip, malignancy, jealousy, war, criticism

Healing Treatment:

I am the extension of the Endless Mind. The Endless Mind never sees an obstruction, ever for It is Omnipotent, Omnipresent and All-Knowing.

Therefore, what's valid for the Endless Mind is also valid for me. I am

completely infused by this Universal Power.

I am one cell in the body of the Endless Mind. Essentially, there can be no real enmity between me and any other cell, ever. There can't be no competition between us, because each of us work in harmony and union, one for the other, consciously or unconsciously. I refuse to misunderstand others and refuse to be misunderstood.

To know all is to forgive all. Therefore, I know that what appears to be hostile – looks, words or actions is only the effort of another to be secure within himself.

I carry the feeling of forgiveness to anyone who wronged me. I refuse to induce suspicion toward those who have not wronged me. I cultivate the expectancy of good in all people and I draw from them the same feelings.

This is the Truth and it is so. I now release this thought into the Endless Mind. I thank the Endless Mind for full manifestation of my desire.

False Belief #6: Rejection ("People reject me.")

This belief causes lack of confidence and comes from the way you were raised by your parents or influenced by your friends, strangers and colleagues.

Correct Thought #6: Self-Confidence ("I know my true worth.")

Removes: Dislocations, fractures, and detached retina. Reverts business failures, failure to attract love and friends, hesitation, suppressed rage, self-deprecation, difficulty to find right work, inspirations and misunderstanding by others

Healing Statement:

I am the extension of the Endless Mind. The Endless Mind never sees an obstruction, ever, for It is Omnipotent, Omnipresent and All-Knowing. Therefore, what's valid for the Endless Mind is also valid for me and I am completely infused by this Universal Power.

There is only One Endless Mind and I am united with IT at every point. Values of The Endless Mind lie in me. I am better, wiser, stronger and more attractive person than I have allowed myself to believe. In fact, I am the only rejecter of myself.

Others see me as I see myself. I have undervalued myself. Others may have caught this thought from the atmosphere. They will now catch the new atmosphere, because I know my true worth.

Therefore, all who meet me know my true worth. Every part of me is strongly united to every other part and to the Universal Power, in mind, body and character.

This is the Truth and it is so.

I now release this thought into the Endless Mind. I thank the Endless Mind for full manifestation of my desire.

Special Variation of Healing Statement for Attracting A Soul Mate

"I am the extension of the Endless Mind. The Endless Mind never sees an obstruction, ever for It is Omnipotent, Omnipresent and All-Knowing.

Therefore, what's valid for the Endless Mind is also valid for me and I am completely infused by this Universal Power.

There is only One Endless Mind and I am united with It at every point.

Infinite Mind's values lie in me. I am better, wiser, stronger and more attractive person than I have allowed myself to believe.

I know that I have believed a lie in thinking that I was ever rejected by anyone. I know that I am greatly desired by the type of man/woman who would fill my ideals. I know that he will never find true and lasting happiness until he finds it in me. He needs me just as truly as I need him. Neither one confers a one-sided benefit upon the other. Each gives and each gets.

The Infinite Knower knows where each of us is today. He is even now moving us across the chessboard of life so that we shall meet, and we shall recognize one another.

I let go of all my tenseness, relinquishing the entire responsibility for the meeting to the Endless Mind. I know that I am not in competition with anyone for this man/woman, and he is not in competition with anyone else for me. He needs me, wants me, loves me, and all these emotions are returned by me.

I now release this situation to the Endless Mind, giving thanks to its completion now, even before I see its manifestation. This is the Truth and it is so.

I thank the Endless Mind for full manifestation of my desire.


False Belief #7: Wrong Action ("Sickness and trouble are natural.") Correct Thought #7: Right Action ("Health and joy are natural.") Removes: All illness, problems, disappointment, sorrow, poverty.

Healing Statement:

I am the extension of the Endless Mind. The Endless Mind never sees an obstruction, ever, for It is Omnipotent, Omnipresent and All-Knowing. Therefore, what's valid for the Endless Mind is also valid for me and I am completely infused by this Universal Power.

The universe is based on laws of perfect action. These laws reflect the

Universe and its intent toward everything IT has ever created.

I am part of that creation and therefore I am intended to profit from the law of the right action.

Only my false belief can hinder the law of right action materializing in me and through me. I now look for the right to come forth. Whenever the wrong manifests I will know it emerges from my false belief.

I will ignore it and carry on with my new thoughts that manifest through the Endless Mind. I surrender myself daily to the Right Action in all my circumstances and life events.

This is the Truth and it is so.

I now release this thought into the Endless Mind. I thank the Endless Mind for full manifestation of my desire.

Note:

Some of you may wonder whether mere recitation of Healing Statements is enough to reach your subconscious mind level.

My answer is yes, as I already pointed out that the subconscious mind always listens and stores all your thoughts and inputs from five senses of sight, hearing, touch, taste and smell.

.

# THE 8-MINUTE STRENGTH & FAT LOSS

Working at maximal intensity for an extended amount of time is physiologically impossible. So if you think that performing tougher workout routines for longer durations will make you shed fat faster, you may want to change your weight loss strategy.

In fact, there is a much more effective way to experience body transformation in much lesser time. Instead of spending hours grinding it out with traditional workout regimes, there is a better and faster way to reap the full fitness benefits by utilizing high intensity movements in short bursts. By doing so, you grant your body frequent recovery periods to prepare for the next round.

Countless studies prove that high intensity training will facilitate in losing body fat fast while retaining maximal muscle mass. High intensity training can also strengthen the cardio vascular system and improve your endurance for high level of intensity training for a longer period of time.

## Chapter 1 What is HIIT?

Fitness enthusiasts who're looking for effective ways to get shredded should know about the term 'HIIT', also known as High Intensity Interval Training. For most people who are unfamiliar with HIIT, they commonly associate it with panting, sweating along with unfathomable amount of burpees.

Perhaps, you've heard that HIIT has to do with performing intense movements, short breaks and breaking an insane amount of sweat. But the truth of the matter is that HIIT is so much more than that.

Yes, there is an element of high intensity as well as of interval training but having said that, most people never perform HIIT workouts correctly. At the end of the day, they might not even get a single HIIT workout in, even though they thought they did. So to clear out the confusion, here is what HIIT truly looks like.

High intensity interval training or HIIT is a very specific type of training technique where you give everything you have during short but fierce spurts of exercise. The bursts are alternated with short and occasionally active periods of recovery as opposed to standing still.

This kind of intense training raises and keeps the heart rate up while burning deep into your fat deposits in less time. You can also get the same benefit when you go for a long run by keeping your heart rate up, also known as Moderate Intensity Steady State Cardio (MISS Training). However, the two are very different, as the results produced vary significantly.

The goal of HIIT is not only to raise your heart rate up and making sure that you perform your training at maximum intensity. And to truly reap the benefits of HIIT, you have to push your efforts to the limit during every burst by keeping your EPOC (Excess Post- Exercise Oxygen Consumption) high.

This is also why each burst is short, ranging anywhere between 20- 90 seconds because even this much time is a lot when you kick the intensity level up to the max.

This key difference separates HIIT from both high intensity and interval training when done on their own. Research shows that all exercise promotes fat burn by burning calories but exercise performed at a higher intensity creates the after-burn effect that burns more calories over time. That is exactly why HIIT is such a hit.

When compared to other types of cardio, HIIT has also been seen to be a more effective means of getting incredibly shredded fast. It is a workout that is beneficial on multiple fronts since it uses both body weight and added weight that not only spike up the heart rate but also tone muscles.

The other thing that makes HIIT work is the element of rest. The training is comprised of intense bursts of activity followed by active recovery, this is where the element of rest comes in. Resting between each set is an essential part of the workout because if you do not take enough time to recover, you will not be able to push yourself to the limit on the next burst.

Since you are performing at an intense level, you are forcing your body to perform something it is neither used to nor comfortable with. Only by pushing through the limits your muscles demand growth. This explains why HIIT can not only burn fat, but also help you retain muscle mass or even grow in mass – In fact, you won't find this benefit by performing long hours of traditional cardio sessions.

To put it simply, HIIT can help you shred body fat, staying lean, improve endurance while adding more muscle mass.

**The Science Behind HIIT**

As seen above, HIIT aims to induce overload. That is to say, by going through strenuous exercise, the body fatigues more significantly in the hope for supercompensation. However, supercompensation can only occur when the training overload is supported by significant recovery. Together, the two components aim to bring about physiological adaptations that lead to increased performance above the baseline.

Think of it like a car engine after a long car trip. Once you have reached your destination, your car engine continues to stay warm until it slowly cools to a resting temperature. The same mechanism occurs happens in the body after a HIIT workout.

Just as a car engine stays warm once it has been turned off, your body's metabolism continues to strive even after the workout is done. This physiological effect is known as excess post exercise oxygen consumption or EPOC.

## The EPOC Effect

Also known as the afterburn effect, EPOC helps burn more calories long after finishing your workout. This occurs when the quantity of oxygen consumed after exercise exceeds that of the pre-exercise level.

During recovery, energy resources need to be replenished, blood needs to be re-oxygenated while circulatory hormones need to be restored. Plus, body temperature needs to return to normal along with the breathing and heart rates. All these physiological reactions require oxygen and so EPOC experiences an increase in calories post exercise as compared to pre exercise.

Now, while EPOC is applicable to most types of intense workouts, research indicates that HIIT is the most effective means to trigger the EPOC effect. This is because when you perfrom your exercises at a higher intensity and demand immediate energy, anaerobic pathways provide the needed ATP at a much faster rate.

This is also the reason why high intensity activity can only be maintained for a brief period of time. So HIIT is effective because high intensity bouts create anaerobically produced ATP and once it is exhausted, it needs to be replenished aerobically.

This also ties in with the fact that EPOC is more affected by the intensity of the workout and not so much by its duration. So even when HIIT workout is done, the body continues to use aerobic energy pathways to replace ATP used up during the session, which boosts the EPOC effect.

The higher the EPOC effect, the more calories you burn at rest and the higher your Resting Metabolic Rate or RER. This spike and recovery pattern is key to making HIIT work flawlessly. Not only does this pattern improve cardiorespiratory endurance but it also allows for greater caloric expenditure during and after the workout when compared to moderate aerobic workouts.

Having said that, it's still crucial to remember that at least 48 hours of recovery time should be allowed between high intensity exercise sessions and should not be performed more than three times a week.

## Is HIIT Right For You?

Since HIIT is all about intensity, you need to be in fairly good health with an elementary level of general and core strength along with mobility. You also need to be aware of your personal physical limitations.

People who want to take on HIIT should be willing to try out a number of different exercises and be knowledgeable about performing these moves not only correctly but safely as well. If you are above the age of 55, then it is recommended that you take on HIIT with a doctor's approval.

HIIT is not recommended for anyone with any orthopedic limitations such as knee, back, or shoulder conditions. Likewise anyone suffering from cardiovascular issues like hypertension and heart palpitations should not take on such an aggressive form of exercise.

## Chapter 2 Benefits of HIIT

Everyone wants the fastest, most efficient way to get in shape and HIIT delivers. As such, the idea of being able to work out for only a short period of time and still have washboard abs sounds like a no brainer. So when you are pressed for time but want to stay lean and healthy, HIIT training is the ideal way to get the job done quickly and effectively.

That said, HIIT is an ideal solution for anyone who does not have the time to exercise for long durations. Individuals on the go, those with hectic schedules or not willing to invest too much time into fitness can benefit, although effort is non-negotiable.

While additional calorie burn, fat loss, muscle gain and improved endurance are a given with HIIT training- and will be discussed in greater details later on, here are some of the most promising benefits HIIT training can offer:

### Improves Oxygen Consumption

In simple terms, oxygen consumption can be described as the ability of the muscles to use oxygen. For non-athletic personnel, typically this is possible only after regularly cycling or running but with HIIT, the benefits can be achieved by anyone and in a much shorter period of time.

HIIT improves the stroke volume which is the volume of blood pumped around the body in one contraction. This volume increases when you exercise given the body's higher need for oxygenated blood.

A study conducted regarding oxygen consumption stated that in a five-week time period, working out four days weekly with 20 minute HIIT workouts led to improved oxygen consumption by almost 9 percent of the subjects. The result is the same as cycling for 40 minutes every day which requires far greater energy consumption.

So HIIT may improve oxygen consumption as much as traditional endurance training, even when you exercise for only half as long.

## Cardiovascular Benefits

In terms of health benefits other than weight loss and improved oxygen consumption, HIIT can provide immense cardiovascular health benefits.

Perhaps the most important thing in this regard is lowering resting heart rate and reducing blood pressure.

While it is well known that extreme training delivers extreme results, most people find it hard to push themselves to an anaerobic zone. HIIT training makes it easier to get into the anaerobic zone as it requires you to perform each bursts with maximum intensity whereby your heart beats faster, you lose your breath more often and then lowering your heart rate during the rest interval that follows. Over time, this training can result in a lower resting heart rate, which also lowers the risk of having heart diseases.

Likewise, HIIT can also help with lowering blood pressure levels as this form of intense exercise can help reduce arterial stiffness. High intensity interval training can also improve endothelial function which is the ability of the arteries to dilate better than moderate intensity training. Good endothelial function is important for blood pressure control and blood vessel health.

Comparative studies have shown that HIIT to be more effective than traditional cardio done at a steady pace in lowering blood pressure readings.

## Helps Reduce Blood Sugar

When done over a period of 12 WEeks, HIIT can also be beneficial for reducing blood sugar levels. Not only does it improve metabolism but also optimizing insulin resistance.

Patients with diabetes are often asked to exercise to bring their blood glucose levels down. Research now shows that HIIT training rapidly improves diabetics' glucose metabolism in muscles and insulin sensitivity in type 2 diabetes.

Intense muscular contractions during HIIT stimulates muscles to take up glucose from the blood to be used as fuel which lowers glucose concentrations. Interestingly, the same also happens whether insulin is present or not, so the approach can also work with people with type 1 diabetes.

## Boosts Metabolism

As mentioned earlier, combining high intensity with interval training brings about EPOC which has the result of speeding the metabolic rate. The effects of this mechanism can be felt for up to 48 hours after a HIIT workout. This means that you will continue to burn fat long after leaving the gym.

Researchers also agree that as compared to jogging or running, HIIT can really push up the metabolic rate. Also, another plus point of this training is that it allows utilization of body fat for energy rather than just carbs alone.

A study concluded that only 2 minutes of high-intensity interval training led to increased metabolism for 24 hours which could easily outweigh the benefits of 30 minutes of jogging.

## Time Saving Features That Require No Equipment

With HIIT you no longer have the excuse of not having sufficient time. In fact, HIIT workouts are doable anywhere from your home to a hotel suite and even outside in the park.

Plus workouts are quick and short, with the longest being no more than 30 minutes at most. Who doesn't have time for that!

Another benefit of HIIT is that it doesn't require any specific equipment helping you save money while providing health benefits at the same time.

## Create Customized Workouts

If you are not up to using weights or machines for your workout, no worries. HIIT can be customized to your individual level and skills.

The most basic workout may use only body weight as the aim is to get your heart rate up and keep it there. You get to pick any kind of exercise which elevates the heart rate and then create an interval workout.

You also get to change your exercises every session which provides an advantage and allows you to not tire or get bored by doing the same thing again and again.

## Challenging And Entertaining

HIIT is a fun and entertaining way to reduce fat and improve overall body health as it allows you to keep changing workouts eradicating the boredom element.

The same also provides a challenge to beginners and newbies by helping them transform and see the changes in their body. It is a challenge to let go of the comfort zone and pursue an exercise that holds massive benefits.

## HIIT Is Efficient

If you have a busy schedule and are unable to work out regularly, HIIT is the thing for you. If you have an event coming up for which you want to look gorgeous, try HIIT as it is more effective than a regular workout and can provide noticeable results much faster.

## Chapter 3 The Essentials of HIIT

HIIT Training can give some amazing results if performed correctly. However, there are a few essentials that you need to consider before starting HIIT. For instance, features like the duration of this routine, the equipment you require and the extent to which you need to go in terms of intensity of the workout are important.

## What Equipment To Use In HIIT?

Beginner HIIT training can be fairly effective with just your body weight, but as you move along, you may want to introduce some equipment into your routines.

HIIT training can be done using an assortment of methods. You can work with anything from a Stairmaster to a bike or treadmill and even incorporate sprinting, bicycle sprints or elliptical workouts.

But whichever machine or activity you choose, you need to do it hard, fast and only stop when you feel that you can't possibly push any further.

A popular choice for HIIT in this regard is a treadmill. It is best to use a curved treadmill since this provides a full body workout. Another common choice for high intensity workouts is the stationary bike to accelerate heart rate and keep it pounding there.

An arm bike is also a good machine to use during high intensity workouts. Working out on this machine requires maximum effort and wrestlers have been using it for building their strength for a long time.

However, if you do not have the budget for all these machines or a gym membership, you can simply get a jump rope. A jump rope will get your heart rate up and keep it there for the duration of the workout.

If you want to follow a somewhat no-equipment HIIT plan, then stick with moves like jumping jacks, sprinting or sprinting in place, and high knees to get your heart going.

**How Intense Should The Workouts Be?**

High intensity workouts are cardio workouts that are aimed at getting the maximum effort in a short period of time. The key is to keep the intensity levels at the maximum.

But for the workout to be effective, you need to determine your own intensity level. For a beginner, the intensity of a HIIT routine will be different from someone who has been doing it for a while. The sets are short in duration, ranging from 20 to 90 seconds but they require full body force. If you feel that you can continue a routine for more than 30 minutes, then chances are that you are not working at maximum intensity.

HIIT is more popular as compared to other methods because it burns calories more rapidly. It has been seen through research that the more intense a workout is, more fat is burnt. Normally, fitness experts judge the intensity level suitable for a person using the RPE scale or the rate of perceived exertion scale.

This scale basically has a 1-10 spectrum, with 10 being the point where you give the workout everything you have got. Every person needs to determine where they stand on this spectrum and try to move to 10 by gradually upping the intensity of their workouts.

**How Restful Should The Rest Periods Be?**

While most people do find this strange, rest periods are imperative in a HIIT workout session. Without rest periods, you cannot get the full benefits of the workout. Once you are done with one set of exercise, your body needs to recover before it can perform the next set.

The mechanism for HIIT is that the body first goes into an anaerobic state during the high intensity workout. During the rest phase, the body is forced to recover to aerobic conditions. This shift between the two conditions consumes a lot of energy and results in fat burning.

The HIIT rest period does not have to be full rest. You can also have an active recovery period, such as a plank or walking in place. The ratio that most fitness experts follow is a one to two ratio. For every one minute of high intensity workout, you have to take a recovery period of 2 minutes.

To see if your workout is going well, you need to see if you can talk and exercise at the same time. If you have the energy left to talk while working out, then there is something that you are not doing quite right.

As you progress and your body becomes used to high intensity workouts, you can make some changes in the sets and rounds of sets. You can either add another set to your workout plan or you can decrease the recovery period between the sets.

To get maximum benefits, make the recovery periods active. For example, for the two minutes recovery time that you get, spend one in a plank and the other in full rest state.

**How Long Should The Workouts Be?**

The duration for a HIIT workout will vary from one person to the next. It also depends on the kind of workout you are doing.

For example, a Tabata session lasts for only 4 minutes. This routine was developed by a Japanese scientist and is very popular among the HIIT group. Normally, a high intensity training session can last for up to 30 minutes.

However, you do not have to work out constantly for 30 minutes. Break up your workout session into working time and recovery time or split the workout into two to three workouts. Make every workout for 6 to 7 minutes and incorporate recovery time in between to make the total duration up to half an hour.

If you do not have recovery time in between, you will most probably get bored of doing the same thing again and again. Plus, overdoing high intensity workouts can be problematic since it may result in injury. As such, you have to plan out your workout properly.

## How Frequently Should You Do HIIT Workouts?

Just like training any of your muscles, you don't want to train chest every single day. So, you should not perform HIIT workouts daily because it is practically impossible to get maximum results by not allowing your body to recover. If you perform high intensity workouts every single day, it can poses the risk of injury.

This can also happen because you are not giving your muscles and the entire body enough time to repair before diving into another wear and tear session. If you are doing too much of it, your mind will also not be on the same track. You are bound to feel fatigue and that will affect the performance in subsequent workout sessions.

It is advisable to perform HIIT two to three times a week. The key is to give your body a one day recovery time between the sessions. For example, if you are doing intense leg workouts, you will not have sufficient energy to work out the very next day. So, keep the next day for rest or do some light yoga instead.

## How To Prevent Muscle Burn During HIIT?

The aim of a HIIT session is to burn fat and not muscle. Therefore, to prevent muscle burn, there are a few things that need to be considered. Firstly, it is absolutely essential to take rest days. These days will give your body and your brain to recharge and prepare for the next workout session.

Another important factor to consider is nutrition. To benefit from any workout, it is important that you're constantly fueled with proper nutrition. You need to take in ample amounts of proteins as they aid in the repair process of the body. Protein supplements are also a great way of preventing muscle burn. They contain amino acids that are then used by the body as building blocks for repairing damaged muscle fibers or to make new ones.

Fitness pros also recommend getting sufficient sleep. Your body heals itself while you sleep. Proper sleep will keep you active for the next workout and it also gives the body some time to repair itself before the next session.

So to reap the maximum benefits of a HIIT workout session, it is imperative to know the basic dynamics of the routine. The duration, intensity and rest periods are all important factors that need to be kept in mind when performing high intensity workouts. Neglecting even one of these factors may pour all your hard work down the drain.

## Chapter 4 HIIT for Fat Loss and Muscle Gain

HIIT is no doubt a great way to melt off those body fat. The workout aims at quick fat burning and the ultimate reduction of fat cells that store fat reserves. But before moving on to the mechanism of fat burning by high intensity workouts or any other methods, you need to understand the mechanism of fat storage in the body.

When you consume food, some of it is used as glucose for energy expenditure. The extra food is stored in the form of glycogen in the liver. This is the reserve food that is used once the glucose levels in the body become low.

Fats and triglycerides are also used by the body for energy and fats provide the largest amount of energy. Extra fat is stored in cells called adipocytes that are abundant in the flank, thighs and the abdomen region. The aim of any exercise is to signal the body burn these reserve carbs and fats.

But before this happens, the body has to exhaust the glucose and triglycerides that are already present in the body. Once those are used up for fuel, the body starts to use the reserve glycogen and fats.

## How Does HIIT Cause Fat Loss?

Metabolism refers to all the processes that take place in the body. These can be of two types.

- Anabolic

These are the reactions in which new products are synthesized using the reactants that are present in the body. These things are often extracted from the food we take in, such as proteins and carbs.

- Catabolic

These reactions are the ones in which something is broken down into smaller particles or for excretion from the body. These reactions may be fat oxidation in which fats are burnt into their respective components. Other than that, catabolic reactions include carb burning and breaking down of larger nutrients into their monomers use these building blocks for making something new.

Both these reactions take place side by side and both need energy to function. This energy comes from burning carbs that are already present in the body.

When a person performs a high intensity workout, their metabolic rate is enhanced. Due to this acceleration of the metabolic rate, reactions in the body also take place at a faster rate. Since more reactions occur and at a faster rate, the fat reserves in the body also start being used up for energy.

With HIIT your metabolism remains in action even in the resting stage; HIIT is much better at enhancing resting metabolism than aerobic exercises. It keeps the resting metabolism going on at a significant rate for 24 hours after the workout, which is just in time for the next workout. Therefore, it keeps the body burning fat during the whole day, even when at rest.

## HIIT And Fat Oxidation

Fat oxidation is the process in which fats are broken down into triglycerides. In cells, oxidation of fat occurs as a result of which triglycerides are produced. These are used for energy provision or they can be stored in the adipose tissue. Since HIIT induces fat oxidation, it ensures that body fat is being broken down instead of getting stored up.

The liver is the only organ in the body that can dispose of cholesterol. When fat reserves build up on the liver, the liver cannot function properly due to pressure exerted on it by the fat concentration. As a result of HIIT, the fat reserves melt which causes the liver to function properly for disposing off cholesterol.

**Increase In Growth Hormone Levels**

HIIT has also shown to increase growth hormone levels. This hormone is also involved in the fat burning mechanism in the body along with enhancing metabolism. In the presence of this hormone, the metabolic rate of the body improves and the efficiency of metabolism is also enhanced significantly.

During high intensity workouts, a chemical is produced in the body called catecholamine. This chemical facilitates fat loss since it mobilizes the stored fat. The fat reserves keep increasing in the body until the previous ones are burnt.

In the presence of this chemical, the fat that is stored in the adipose tissue is mobilized so that it can be used as fuel for energy. The primary source for fuel in the body is carbohydrates so the body has to produce some kind of chemical to make the fats available for fuel.

**How Does HIIT Build Muscle Mass?**

HIIT is also responsible for building muscle mass. This is because HIIT builds endurance and causes more blood flow with better contractility to the muscles. The blood carries oxygen and nutrients to all parts of the body. After high intensity workouts, more oxygen is taken to the muscles. This results in oxidative respiration in the muscle.

Anaerobic conditions cause the production of lactic acid in muscles. This is why the muscles feel fatigued and they get sore. If more oxygen is taken to the muscles, aerobic conditions persist and oxidation process occurs. As a result, you build more muscle mass in the long run.

Moreover, blood also takes nutrients to the muscles. These nutrients are essential for the muscle growth and development, especially the proteins. Proteins can be used as energy source for growth of the muscles. Also, they are great for repair.

Every time you work out, muscle wear and tear takes place which has to be treated by the body. Proteins play a role in this process and they repair the muscle fibres that have been damaged during intense workouts. Also, they make new muscle fibres using amino acid as building blocks. These amino acids are used for making muscle proteins called actin and myosin which are responsible for muscle contraction and relaxation.

## Metabolism And Muscle Mass

HIIT increases the rate of metabolism in the muscles in active stage and keeps metabolic activities going on even in the resting stage. In the anabolic reactions, new products are made for muscles. In this process, muscle mass is also built. Since high intensity workouts keep the anabolic activities going on for 24 hours following the workout, they ensure that muscle synthesis is taking place at all times.

As such, high intensity workouts are great for burning fat since they increase the metabolic rate and also increase the fat oxidation rate in the body. Plus, it also reduces appetite and increases fat mobility by increasing the amount of catecholamine. Along with fat loss, high intensity workouts are also responsible for increasing lean muscle mass which is a great way for people to get their dream body.

## Chapter 5 HIIT for Endurance

To build endurance, you don't have to spend hours of your daily life training and doing intense exercises. HIIT is a great way for building endurance since it focuses on the major endurance- building points in the body.

One of the main elements of endurance is cardiovascular performance. This refers to the way your heart works and the subsequent working of the circulatory system in response to heart's pumping. The functioning of the heart can be measured by three determinants.

1.      Heart Rate

This is the rate of your heart beating per minute. The more your heart beats in a minute, the more blood is pumped to the body and the faster your body moves towards endurance.

2.      Stroke Volume

This refers to the blood amount that is pumped every time the heart beats. Since there is a direct relationship between the stroke volume and endurance, a higher stroke volume is beneficial for the body.

3.      Contractility

This refers to the force with which your heart pumps blood to the body. The stronger the force, the farther the blood travels. If contractility is higher, an individual has more blood flowing to the exercising muscles. This blood is laden with oxygen and nutrients that are then utilized by the skeletal muscles for strength and repair.

## How Is Endurance Built?

Endurance is not only a measurement of how hard your heart is pumping blood. It also refers to the amount of oxygen that can be delivered to your muscles. This variable is called VO2. This variable depends on the factors mentioned above as well as on the amount of oxygen that is extracted from the blood that enters the muscles. Not all the oxygen that is taken to the muscles by the blood is taken by the muscles. The oxygen has to be extracted first and the more oxygen extraction capacity the muscles have, more oxygen they will receive.

Another factor that contributes to endurance is the mitochondrial density. It is common knowledge that mitochondria is the power house of the cell. What this means is that it is involved in the production of energy in the form of ATP. This energy is produced through different cycles that take place in the mitochondria. The higher the mitochondrial density, the more energy is produced for the consumption of the body.

## How Does HIIT Build Endurance?

HIIT builds endurance by working on all the variables that are mentioned above. It enhances the stroke volume for ensuring a greater amount of blood flow to the skeletal muscles. Moreover, it also has an effect on contractility and increases the pumping force of the heart.

As far as mitochondrial density is concerned, HIIT is a great alternative to aerobic exercises for increasing your mitochondrial density. If there are more mitochondria is the body, more energy production takes place and that gives the muscles more endurance.

Another way in which HIIT induces endurance is by increasing the number of enzymes present in the mitochondria. As mentioned above, energy is produced in the mitochondria through different cycles. In all the steps of these cycles, different enzymes act on the substrate to form a product. These enzymes have their distinctive activities that are essential for energy production. HIIT leads to an increase in these enzymes and these enzymes then further increase the endurance in skeletal muscles.

When you perform HIIT, it shifts the signalling pathway in the body from a slower to a faster one. For breakdown of nutrients and extraction of energy from them, the mitochondria are activated through a 'switch' in the body called PGCa. During high intensity exercises, the signalling pathway for activation of this switch is a lot faster. As a result of that, the enzymes' activity is enhanced and the mitochondrial density is also increased.

## HIIT and VO2

As mentioned above, the VO2 levels in the blood determine how much oxygen is getting to the skeletal muscles and other parts of the body. HIIT has shown to significantly enhance VO2 levels in the body and enhances stroke volume. Since the stroke volume is enhanced through high intensity workouts, more blood gets sent to the body every single time the heart contracts. This is a good thing for the skeletal muscles since they start getting more blood.

The circulatory system of the body is responsible for transport of nutrients and oxygen to the muscles and other organs. When the skeletal muscles get more blood, they also get more oxygen and nutrients. This is essential for proper growth and functioning of the muscles.

Using this oxygen, they can respire and release energy using the mitochondria present in them. At the same time, the amino acids in the nutrients are further used for repair and for synthesis of new proteins that are needed for the muscles.

High intensity workouts also increase cardiac contractility which refers to the force with which the heart pumps blood. As the pumping force is increased, the blood reaches all muscles and organs of the body. When skeletal muscles get more blood, they build up endurance. It is due to this excessive endurance that the individual has shorter recovery time and can perform much better in gym sessions.

## HIIT Builds Endurance In Skeletal Muscles

High intensity workouts also build endurance in skeletal muscles. When you perform these exercises, the vasculature of the skeletal muscle is changed. The vasculature refers to the size and number of blood vessels that are present in the area. Due to these workouts, tiny blood vessels become apparent in the skeletal muscles.

They enhance the heart stroke by sending more blood to the heart. The muscles, when contracting, send blood back to the left ventricle of the heart. If more blood is being sent to the heart, it means more blood is being oxygenated too. Thus, heart stroke is enhanced and more blood is sent back to the body in oxygenated form. This increases the amount of nutrients getting to the muscles.

HIIT also enhances endurance by increasing the strength of muscle fibres. The muscles fibres are made up on proteins. In high intensity workouts, the blood circulation is enhanced and more of these proteins are being made using the amino acids present in the blood. This enhances the flexibility of the muscle fibres and makes them stronger.

## Motor Units And HIIT

The skeletal muscle fibres have something called motor units. These units are important for signalling in the muscles and for building endurance. High intensity workouts increase the number of motor units present in the body. This can aid in two things.

•        If more motor units are present in the skeletal muscles, then muscle coordination improves and the person has better endurance.

•        Motor units also help to reduce the fatigue time for exercises. As such, anyone with enhanced motor units does not tend to get tired quickly.

## Does HIIT Affect Qmax?

Qmax is referred to the maximum amount of blood that your heart can pump to the body in a minute. It has been seen in studies that high intensity workouts have little or no significant effect on Qmax. On the contrary, low intensity workouts such as aerobic workout plans are great for increasing Qmax.

Therefore, HIIT takes cardiovascular pathways to increase endurance. It increases the density of mitochondria in the cells along with enhancing the functioning of mitochondrial enzymes. Furthermore, it strengthens the muscle fibres by giving them more proteins for repair and strength. High intensity workouts also increase endurance by overall increasing the VO2 max and by keeping the oxygen volume in the blood high at all times, for transfer to the skeletal muscles.

## Chapter 6 Common Mistakes When Doing HIIT

HIIT is, beyond doubt, a very effective workout but to get results, it needs to be done correctly. Most people are not used to pushing themselves as hard as necessary for HIIT especially for a workout that is as short as 7- 10 minutes because it is extremely uncomfortable.

That is why many people often start making mistakes during their workouts which can easily sabotage their efforts and diminish their results. Here is a look at some of the most common mistakes to avoid when doing HIIT.

### Opting For Longer Workouts

Essentially, a HIIT session can last anywhere from four to twenty minutes, or thirty minutes if stretched to the maximum. If someone is able to push it beyond that, then that is not an achievement.

It is a common error to go for longer sessions during HIIT. The whole point is to push your body to the maximum limit during high intensity periods. This will automatically make your sessions shorter as the body will be too exhausted to work anymore.

### Not Warming Up

HIIT training can be tough and strenuous, especially for beginners who are not yet ready to use their body's maximum potential during their workout sessions. Even those who are physically fit and active need to warm up before they start with their HIIT training.

It is a common mistake to directly hit the gym and get going with the session. This will reduce the effects that you are trying to achieve. Without a warm up, the body will not be able to give it's all during the high intensity intervals.

## Choosing Complex And Complicated Movements

Experts say that with subsequent sessions of workouts, the body can get too tired to perform a complex movement. During your first session, a complicated movement might not seem that bad at all. But after repeated movements, the body and brain could be overstrained, increasing the chances of an injury such as sprains or falls.

Instead, it is advised to choose movements for HIIT workouts that are easier to perform, without having to put too much thought into which body part goes where and which muscle to stretch more than the other.

Apart from choosing complex movements, another common mistake is not perform the easy ones correctly. As simple as a movement might be, unless you are performing it right, it is not going to be effective.

It is always good to give your mind and body a chance to master a movement first before you start training faster.

Not Paying Attention To 'Recovery' Intervals

This is one of the most common mistakes during HIIT to reduce the resting or recovery intervals in an attempt to make it 'tougher'. This is the wrong idea.

The recovery period is as important as the high intensity interval, if not more. This is the period where the muscles pay off what is called an 'oxygen debt'. They receive the oxygen that they were deprived off as the workout proceeded and led up to their fatigue. Once they get the oxygen back, they can work just as hard in the next high intensity period. If ample recovery time is not taken, then muscles are only partially ready for the next hard work.

## Not Being 'Intense' Enough

By high intensity during HIIT training, it is meant that you should be extremely breathless, the heart thumping loudly against your chest and your body and brain both screaming that you cannot push any further. If this does not happen to you during your high intensity intervals, you are making the same mistake as many others: not going hard enough.

You need to push yourself to the point where you physically and mentally reach a point beyond which you know you cannot go on. Only then will your HIIT workout be a success.

Most HIIT training sessions involve movements and exercises that are natural and easy. They make the workout more effective and also reduce the chances of an injury. Lifting weights can also be a part of high interval sessions but these weights should not be too heavy. The easier they are to lift, the better.

## Diet And Clothing Matter

As good as it might look, wearing clothes that are too tight are only going to bother you during the workout. It is important to invest in proper gym clothes that are made of a breathable material, do not trap sweat against your skin and leave you itchy. It is also necessary to wear proper trainers for your sessions.

In terms of nutrition, first and foremost is to stay hydrated! Drink ample water well before your workout session starts because it's about to get sweaty!

There are many protein shakes available, which can be used. Otherwise a good fibre and lean protein meal works just as fine. Having said that, it is best to be done eating at least an hour before your session. It is a common error to eat right before working out and not pay attention to what you eat either. Fruits and vegetables just before working out are not going to be very helpful.

## Not Staying Determined Enough

The last thing your body needs to hear is 'You can't do it!' Yet it hears this a lot during HIIT training. HIIT can be very tough and demanding. It can make the body feel more exhausted than ever.

So it is common to give up. It will feel hard and impossible, and the negative thinking will only make it worse. But sticking to it will allow you to reap some great benefits.

## Doing HIIT Too Often

Boasted by the great outcome and result of HIIT training can lead to the mistake of over doing it such as, trying to do it every day. This is not good for the muscles at all. The maximum frequency of a HIIT session should not be more than twice or thrice a week. This is to allow ample recovery time to the body so that it is all set for the next round.

This is primarily why many people have begun to prefer this over long everyday sessions of low intensity workouts. It does not demand too much time from their busy routines.

## Choosing The Wrong Timing

Randomly choosing half an hour in the week for HIIT workout is a big mistake. The sessions need to be timed properly. Having a session right after you eat or just before bed is a bad idea.

In fact, the sooner in the day you train, the better. Taking a good but light breakfast early in the morning, an hour before the HIIT session is the best way to go about it. This way your fat reserves will be targeted better. It will also prepare your body to burn the calories you will be munching up throughout the day.

As a matter of fact, working out early and before going to work will also maximize your performance there, as the concentration and productivity will be at its best.

## Chapter 7 The Best Diet for HIIT

To benefit from any workout plan to the fullest, it is imperative to have a suitable diet plan, complementing the workout sessions. For HIIT, it is essential to have a diet that is rich in proteins and has sufficient carbs. This ensures that you have enough energy to exercise intermittently without giving in to fatigue. Along with that, an adequate amount of water is also essential for the success of a HIIT workout.

## Pre-Workout Nutrition

HIIT workouts involve short yet extensive workout sessions, which is why it is very important for the pre-workout diet to be high in energy. The human body works all day long and is busy in the processes of muscle-building and repair.

Pre-workout nutrition refers to the diet that you should take about 4 hours before the workout session. If the pre-workout nutrition is planned strategically, it gives the body ample time and energy to recover and make new muscles.

About 4 hours prior to your workout, it is important to take in sufficient amounts of carbohydrates and proteins. Carbs are the body's major source of energy and they give the body that ultimate fuel which is needed to drive a workout. Proteins, on the other hand, are coupled with carbs for repair and muscle building.

The carb intake should be moderate enough to not overload the body but energize it enough for the workout. Some good pre- workout food options include:

• Dried fruit such as almonds or cashew nuts

• Plain Yoghurt (Preferably, a blend of yoghurt, fruits and some veggies in form of a smoothie)

• Protein powder and Whole wheat toast

• A banana and some strawberries or a smoothie

These meals are a great way to energize the body for the workout by giving it the extra energy it requires. Just an hour or so before the actual workout, the body is in need of a 'boost' of energy. This comes from carbohydrates so the meal plan immediately before the workout needs to be rich in carbohydrates. Some good pre-workout meal options include:

• A bowl of fruit

• A nut energy bar

• Peanut butter toast

Then, just half an hour before the workout, take in a scoop of whey protein. This is important to reduce the recovery time for the body in case of muscle fatigue or any energy loss. Proteins are the ultimate muscle building sources of the body and when the body needs repair, they are at the front.

**Post Workout Nutrition**

Likewise, after you are done with such an intense workout, it is important to make up for what the body has lost. Firstly, the body has lost its glycogen reserve, which is the form in which glucose is stored in the body. Secondly, during the workout process, the muscles are also broken down. The main nutrient required for their repair is protein.

As such, the post workout diet plan should have more proteins.

Immediately after a HIIT workout session, it is not possible to fix yourself a proper meal so you can go for quick fixes that have high protein content. Some options include:

- A Protein shake

- A slice of white bread

- Soy milk and 2 spoons of jelly

These foods are to be taken in before the actual meal for the day or night. You can take this half an hour after the workout. The proper meal after a HIIT workout should be rich in carbs and proteins both, since both are needed. Carbohydrates are needed for glucose, a part of which will be stored as glycogen in the liver again.

On the other hand, proteins are needed for repair of worn out muscles. It has been seen thorough research that the best combination of proteins and carbs is in a 1:3 ratio. After you have finished you session, make sure that you have a proper meal in the 2 hours following your workout session.

Proteins need to be included since they are involved in building up muscles. The amino acids present in your diet are the building blocks used to repair damaged muscle cells. Different cells in the body are involved in the process of using amino acids to make new muscle fibers or to damage the ones that have been severed during intense workouts.

Proteins present in milk products are quite beneficial for the muscle health so snacks for HIIT diet plan are normally scoops of whey protein or casein protein.

- Rice with veggies and chicken

- Pasta and salad (add meat sauce for taste)

- A cup of mixed green salad and some salmon

- A cup of green beans and salmon

It is also important to incorporate some healthy fats into your post-workout meal. This is because fats aid in reducing inflammation that often occurs as a result of high intensity workouts. Inflammation, if it prevails, can hinder the exercising process for subsequent days so it is essential to deal with it from day one.

Along with food, it is important to make up for the water lost during the workout session. Keep drinking water throughout the day, till you go to bed. When you exercise, a lot of water is lost in the form of sweat. This needs to be replaced since a hydrated body sees quicker results in terms of exercise.

**3 Day Meal Ideas**

As mentioned above, it is absolutely imperative for a good diet plan to complement a workout session for the exercise plan to yield results. A 3 day meal plan with three main courses of the day along with 2 snacks is given below.

Day 1:

Breakfast

- 2 Whole eggs

- 1 slice low fat cheese

- 2 slices low fat turkey bacon

- 2 slices whole wheat bread

Morning Snack

A cup of berries or a handful of walnuts

Lunch

- Spinach

- 5 oz. shrimp

- Half a cup of dried oatmeal

- A table spoon of salad dressing

Mid-day Snack

- A table spoon of peanut butter

- Half a cup of cottage cheese

Dinner

- Barbeque chicken with natural BBQ sauce

- Whole wheat break

- Cabbage dressing

- 5 oz. kale

Day 2 Breakfast

- An English muffin (whole wheat)

- 3 slices of turkey bacon
- Breakfast sandwich with eggs and a slice of cheese

## Morning Snack

- A cup of cottage cheese
- Half a cup of berries

## Lunch

- 6 oz. chicken breast
- A cup of zucchini sliced well

## Mid-day snack

- A scoop of whey protein
- Handful of any dried fruit

## Dinner

- A large baked potato
- Grilled salmon
- Half a cup cheese and a table spoon of Greek yoghurt
- Salt and hot sauce for taste

Day 3 Breakfast

- 3 whole eggs

- Omelet made with reduced-fat cheese and onions

Morning snack

- A cup of spinach

- 2 spoons of salad dressing with olive oil and vinegar

Lunch

- A cup of broccoli chopped well

- A table spoon of salad dressing with olive oil and vinegar

- 8 oz. of chicken breast

Mid-day snack

- Peanut butter on a whole-wheat toast

Dinner

- Canned tuna sandwich

- Half a cup of Green yoghurt

- Celery stalk chopped well with chopped onions

It is only by consuming ample amount of required nutrients that you can benefit from your workouts. If the pre-workout meals and the post-workouts meals are not sufficiently loaded with the right nutrients, you will feel fatigued in no time and it will also decrease the stamina of the body.

Coupled with this meal plan, it is important to drink 8 to 10 glasses of water every single day to keep hydrated. More water equals a better working metabolism which is helpful for a successful workout.

## Chapter 8 Supplements for HIIT

No matter which workout you are following, most need to couple proper diet with supplements to get the maximum benefits. These supplements are needed for that extra boost of energy and for initiating the repair process in the body. Several supplements are especially suited for HIIT, as they work best for high intensity exercises.

### Greens Supplement

Greens Supplement is a great method for increasing strength and power. It gives the user more strength, which is an important factor in high intensity workouts.

When your body undergoes intense workouts, it starts to accumulate acid. This can slow down performance and cause fatigue. During exercise, the body goes into anaerobic state. When the body respires in the absence or limited amount of oxygen, it produces lactic acid.

Due to the accumulation of acid, the pH begins to drop. This makes the working mechanisms in the muscles stop. As a result of all this, the person feels fatigued and does not have the strength require for the next workout session.

Green supplements have alkaline properties that cancel out the acidity in the muscles. So they can be beneficial in increasing the body's power and in reducing fatigue for maximum performance.

### Creatine Monohydrate

There has been extensive research on creatine. It has been used in many sports supplements since the first discovery of its benefits. Not only does this supplement increase the performance ability, it also increases the lean muscle mass in the body.

The body needs to maintain homeostasis, which is the state of the body in which every factor is well-regulated. Creatine acts as a pH buffer, keeping the pH of the body regulated at all times.

This ensures that the muscles are present in the right pH conditions for maximum overall performance. Plus, creatine lets you enjoy more reps without getting tired or stripped of energy.

Another reason why Creatine is suitable for HIIT training is due to its ability to ensure faster recovery. In HIIT training session, it is a must to include recovery periods. When a person recovers at a faster rate, they can perform better in the gym and reap the maximum benefits of their workouts.

Creatine is also involved in increasing the number of satellite cells that are present in the body. These cells help to increase muscle mass by linking amino acids together for formation of new proteins. More muscle mass is directly proportional to more workouts and better results.

**Caffeine**

It should not come as a surprise that caffeine is helpful in increasing alertness in the body. It is responsible for making you more focused and alert during workouts and enhancing performance. Excessive amounts of caffeine can be harmful so it is important to determine your tolerance and make your daily intake according to that.

It is recommended to take 300 grams maximum, of caffeine before an intense workout. This will give you a surge of energy and keep you focused on the workout.

Caffeine activates the sympathetic nervous system, which is activated when the body is in a state of alertness. In this system, the hormone epinephrine is secreted and induces the breakdown of glycogen present in the muscles. Along with that, it also oxidizes fatty acids in skeletal muscles. Both these processes result in energy production that is later utilized for high intensity workouts.

So, caffeine can increase endurance in the body and keep the body in a high-energy state at all times.

## L-Carnitine L-Tartarate

Both of these are amino acids that are not commonly present in the body in large amounts. The body has 20 major amino acids that are all present in the L confirmation. L-Carnitine is an uncommon amino acid that has to be taken from external sources since it is not readily present in the body.

This amino acid aids in fat burning by mobilizing the fats present in the body for energy. Along with that, it also reduces the recovery time after a long workout. If you normally take two days off after a HIIT workout session, with the use of this supplement, you will be able to reduce the recovery time to one day. This gives you more time to work out and have a lot more endurance.

L-Carnitine is also involved in increasing glycogen reserves in the muscles. When carbs are taken in, the body uses some of it to form glucose and the excess is stored in the body in form of glycogen. This can be broken down for use when body is in need of energy. By increasing the muscle reserves of glycogen, this supplement ensures that muscles have energy whenever it is required.

Plus, this supplement also prevents the formation of free radicals. Free radicals are the by-products produced as a result of different chemical processes taking place in the body and can significantly harm the body in the long run.

During exercise, muscle tissues are damaged due to wear and tear. L-Carnitine keeps the muscles protected from tissue damage so that there is lesser fatigue. In addition, the use of this supplement also reduces muscle soreness and keeps you energized for the next round of workouts.

Taking about 3 grams of this supplement everyday can give the person following a HIIT workout plenty of benefits.

## Betaine

Betaine is a modified form of the amino acid glycine, which occurs naturally in the body. It is also present in many foods including beet, shellfish and spinach. So while it is likely that you are taking some of this supplement in your diet chances are that it may not be enough.

Betaine can form creatine in the body by donating methyl group. And as mentioned above, creatine has plenty of benefits for anyone who works out. Betaine, on its own, also has significant effects on the wellness of skeletal muscles. It keeps lactate levels low and removes this acid and keeps the body energized.

An addition, it increases the rate of protein synthesis in muscle cells. As more proteins are made, more energy is provided to the muscles. Since proteins are involved in body's natural repair mechanism, their ample amount is essential for reducing recovery time.

A study showed that betaine can also lower exhaustion levels. Most athletes and individuals who work out frequently drink water to stay hydrated and reduce exhaustion. When coupled with betaine, water can reduce exhaustion by a factor of 40 times more.

## Citrulline

Citrulline is a supplement that plays a role in synthesizing nitric oxide in the body. Nitric oxide is very important for regulating blood flow to muscles and other organs and can enhance blood flow to the muscles.

Blood contains oxygen and nutrients for the wellness and strength of the body. As more blood flows to muscles, more nutrients are present for the muscles to extract energy. Also, in presence of ample oxygen, the muscles can respire aerobically and have lesser production of lactic acid. This contributes to lessened fatigue and more energy.

Citrulline malate also contributes to fat loss. In normal HIIT sessions, the rate of fat loss is 1.2%. However, with usage of Citrulline malate, the fat loss percentage goes up to 2.3%.

Citrulline, when used as citrulline malate also acts as a buffer for ammonia. It counteracts the effects of lactic acid on the body by cancelling out the acidity and increasing the ph. Taking up to 6 grams of citrulline about an hour before exercise can keep the body energized.

All these supplements complement high intensity workouts and make their results much better. Taking controlled amounts of these supplements ensures utmost performance, shorter recovery times and higher energy levels.

## Conclusion

To sum up, whether your goal is fat loss, muscle gain or athletic performance, HIIT can help you achieve all these goals.

You will continue to get results as long as you do the workouts correctly which means building in rest and recovery between the sessions. Pair it up with a good diet and supplements to boost performance and see your body transform with the shortest, most effective workouts out there.

Made in the USA
Monee, IL
06 October 2020

44152677R00100